SIT, STAY, HEAL

What Dogs Can Teach Us About Living Well

DR. RENEE ALSARRAF

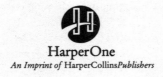

HarperOne

An Imprint of HarperCollins*Publishers*

Excerpt on pages 189–190 from DeMarco, Jerry, "Maywood Police Dog Helps Lead Investigators Toward Hit-Run Killer," *Hackensack Daily Voice*, September 28, 2017, https://dailyvoice.com/new-jersey/hackensack/police-fire/maywood -police-dog-helps-lead-investigators-toward-hit-run-killer/722757/.

HarperCollins books may be purchased for educational, business, or sales promotional use. For information, please email the Special Markets Department at SPsales@harpercollins.com.

FIRST EDITION

Designed by Bonni Leon-Berman

Illustrations on pages 1, 139, and 237 © Shutterstock. All other illustrations from Noun Project.

Library of Congress Cataloging-in-Publication Data has been applied for.

ISBN 978-0-06-321522-1

22 23 24 25 26 LSC 10 9 8 7 6 5 4 3 2 1

To all those who have struggled but made it through
thanks to four legs, a wagging tail, and a warm, wet nose

I have found that when you are deeply
troubled, there are things you get from the
silent devoted companionship of a dog that
you can get from no other source.
—*Doris Day*

Scars are beautiful when we see
them as glorious reminders that we
courageously survived.
—*Lysa TerKeurst*

CONTENTS

Introduction — 1

1 Daisy — 7

2 Bentley — 31

3 Cosmo — 53

4 Dickens, Drummer, and Newton — 69

5 Newton, Part Two — 95

6 Bogart — 111

7 Sasha — 139

8 Franny and Lucky — 163

9 Newton, Part Three — 199

10 Dusty and Callie — 219

Conclusion — 237

Author's Note — 239

Acknowledgments — 241

INTRODUCTION

For the past twenty-nine years, I have worked as a veterinary oncologist. Basically, I treat animals with cancer, primarily dogs and cats, but sometimes an occasional ferret, rabbit, bird, or guinea pig.

People always ask me, "How can you do what you do?" They think cancer in animals is too sad to be a full-time job. They are surprised to hear me say I experience much more happiness than sadness. I consult on cases, I provide chemotherapy, I offer radiation therapy, and I might even recommend surgery. I try to give pet parents realistic hope, another summer or perhaps a few years of good quality time. It is an emotionally draining profession, yet it fills me right back up.

Veterinary patients don't speak to us in words, and so veterinarians use empathy—along with laboratory tests—to find out what's ailing them, and assist them in recovery. Even without words, animals make their feelings known: wagging their tails, giving us kisses, or perhaps growling and baring their teeth. When I can make them feel better it makes me feel better. In fact, it makes me feel joy.

Pets are amazing. Indeed, the word "pet" seems inadequate to describe the special role and deep bond that animals have with their human families. They provide unconditional love when the world feels harsh. We rely on them and even lean on them.

I am fortunate enough to see this human-animal bond in its deepest forms. The power of that bond transcends money, age, and race, and it is without judgment. In some instances, a relationship with a pet may be the only circumstance in which a person feels completely comfortable and loved. There is no shame with an animal, no reason to put on a front. Our four-legged companions accept us as we are, and understand much more than we generally give them credit for.

Some people, however, do not know this bond. Or maybe they don't understand it. Or perhaps they haven't allowed themselves to feel it. Such non–animal people will chastise the devoted pet owner, asking: "How can you spend that kind of money to treat a dog's cancer when you could just get another dog?" Sadly, I have been asked that question numerous times. But animal people understand the truth—our pets are not replaceable; they are not appliances. They're living, breathing, innocent beings who fill a role in our lives, in *my* life.

In the veterinary world, happy dogs go right on being happy when they're first diagnosed. They chew on their bones, bark at the mail carrier, and continue to try to sneak up on the sofa even if they are not supposed to be up on furniture. It is their human family who struggles to deal with the emotions of their pet's condition.

I've sat with many families, counseling them through their love and their grief focused on the mortality of their beloved animal. Their pets never understand why their human is so sad. We're told that we're different from animals—some would even say superior to them. We have a conscience, and we can "think" as well as feel. Perhaps, though, we could take a cue from the four-legged among us. All cats and dogs live in the moment, carefree. They do not waste the present, worried about what might happen in the future. Or how much longer they have to live. We spend a lot of time on the what-ifs, fretting about potential outcomes. I can fret with the best of them. But when has fretting ever really helped us? Can't say it's helped me.

As much as I would like to emulate my animal patients' ability to live in the moment, sometimes that moment is really hard to take. I say that as the car pulls up to let me out at the cancer treatment center. It's a large gray building, bustling with doctors and nurses and support staff. I am not here to work. Today, I am the patient.

That's right: I'm a veterinary oncologist with metastatic

cancer. I'm the animal cancer doc with a diagnosis of my own, which is why I've come to the large gray building. Now it is my time to go through what so many before me have gone through: the *C* word.

I hate the name of my disease. I work to treat cancer every day, and yet when it comes to the diagnosis for myself, I can only call it the *C* word. Dysfunctional? Perhaps. But I detest the word "cancer." It produces instant anxiety and fear in people, and I am no exception. Having this disease has felt like a sucker punch, one that I never, ever expected.

I am not "owning" the struggle. It is not anything that I've asked for, but I will fight it with all that I've got. Now that I face this diagnosis myself, I will approach the battle relentlessly, wholly. I don't like to need help, and I'm not good at asking for it. However, I know I'll need it along the way, as will my family. When I slip off my mental train tracks, I have asked my friends to prop me back up. I'm supposed to be the mom who quizzes her son before big tests at school. The mom who guides him through his college applications. But if I'm sick from treatment, I won't be able to play that role. Will he have to take care of me? Will he pity me? Be ashamed of me?

I'm prepared for any battle as long as I have hope. If I receive devastating news, at least I'll know that in the too-little time I've had here on Earth, I've tried to make my part of it a better place. I've loved my child and my husband

4

wholeheartedly. And I will always cherish my friends. I am extremely grateful to have been able to work in the field that I do. I have learned so much from my animal patients over these years. I've laughed with their owners, cried with their owners, and loved giving families more quality time with their beloved animals. But now I'm hoping for just a little more time of my own.

1

DAISY

It has been a stressful mom morning. My husband, Mike, has taken off much earlier. Lucky man. I am left with a high school boy whose last desire is to get out of bed and a dog who decided to get into the garbage that my dear son was supposed to have taken out last night. I frantically clean up while shouting for Peter to get ready to leave for school before he is marked tardy—again. I drive into work with a white-knuckle grip on the steering wheel.

Finally, I make it to work, a bit crabby, a bit stressed, but here. My 9:00 a.m. appointment slot is a new case. By 9:15 a.m. I'm getting antsy: Where's the appointment? I hate to run late. It stresses me, or, I should say, I *allow* it to stress me, because a late client potentially can put me behind schedule for the entire day. Just as I go up front to the waiting room to check, in walks a smiling blond woman with her hands full. She's a bit disheveled, but happy and doing the best she can, pushing what I initially thought was a large metal stroller, struggling to get the device over the doorframe. On second glance, I see that it's not a stroller but a wheelchair for her nine-year-old child, Kathy. The girl is held in place by safety belts. Tugging at the end of a leash is a panting and eager eleven-year-old cocker spaniel, dressed in a blue princess dress, like Elsa from *Frozen*.

Daisy, the canine Elsa look-alike, was diagnosed with cancer last week. Her family, the Johnsons, had noticed lumps under the cocker's neck—enlarged lymph nodes. Her regular veterinarian took samples from them, which came back from the pathology laboratory as malignant, or cancerous. Mrs. Johnson arrives at this appointment with the biopsy report, blood work, a copy of Daisy's medical records, and chest X-rays in hand. How she balances carrying everything, while pushing her daughter and holding on to Daisy's leash, is impressive. Daisy has lymphoma, the most common form of cancer that a dog can get. But Daisy doesn't appear to have a care in the world. She is wagging her stubby tail so much that her entire rear is wagging with it. She is sniffing the edges of the small exam room that we enter on a mission to find out who was there before her, and with the eager hope of finding a morsel of a dog biscuit in some corner.

I lift Daisy onto the table for a physical examination. I must admit, I've never done a physical on anyone dressed as Elsa, especially an Elsa who tries to lick me on my face. Silly, sweet dog. In examining the cocker, I notice that all ten of her peripheral lymph nodes are enlarged and that she has a bit of a heart murmur. In Daisy's records, it shows that she has had this murmur since puppyhood, but a prior ultrasound of her heart tells me there are no structural issues. Thankfully, the murmur is of no concern.

I place Daisy back on the ground. She's a bit heavy and certainly fills out her dress. I go through the disease process and multiple treatment options with Mrs. Johnson. Chemotherapy is the best route for treating this type of cancer. We can't cure this disease, but chemotherapy typically can put the cancer in a remission and give Daisy a good quality of life for a year or so. Remission for this dog means that all her lymph nodes would go back to normal. Though we could get rid of all clinical evidence of cancer, eventually the cancer cells will become resistant to the drugs, and then the lymphoma will return. Treatment requires frequent visits to the vet hospital, which can be expensive. We discuss three different protocols, all varying based on how many treatments are needed, the prognosis with each, and the costs associated. Prednisone is a steroid pill that can help slow down the course of lymphoma for a couple of months. This is highly recommended for those pet parents who choose not to treat with chemotherapy. I try never to judge or second-guess whether a family elects to treat their pet with chemotherapy. A lot goes into that decision: the flexibility of the pet parent's schedule for coming in, the costs for the tests and the medications, the family's level of tolerance for side effects. In human medicine, more often than not, we are given one treatment path by the physician that we follow, often blindly. Treatment in veterinary medicine is much more of a personal choice.

"If Daisy is doing well, would it be okay to miss a few treatments?" Mrs. Johnson asks with a knitted brow. I can see the wheels turning in her head.

"It is not ideal," I tell her. "Everyone has things that come up—a vacation, a snowstorm—that's understandable and happens to us all. But to keep the cancer at bay, it's best to try to stay on schedule as much as possible."

"Well, maybe I could move some things around," she says, looking down at the floor. "Sometimes we have to go to the children's hospital for a few weeks."

"It is not easy," I say, trying to reassure her. "It's a lot. We'd work around your schedule as best we can."

It would be understandable if the Johnson family opts to limit treatment to the prednisone. They have a lot on their plate, taking care of Kathy, their adopted special-needs daughter. She is unable to speak but uses some sign language. The family feeds their daughter through a gastric tube, a tube directly into her stomach, as she cannot eat by mouth. Kathy watches me intently with her dark eyes, then furtively looks away when I look at her. She glances back with a big smile that lights up her whole, beautiful face. And to think I had been stressed over morning traffic, over being late.

When I was first told of my diagnosis, I felt like someone had pulled the rug out from under me. I still feel that way, and it's an empty, horrifying feeling. I replay that day over and over in my head.

It was 7:00 p.m., July 3. It had been a long, busy day at the clinic, and I hadn't had time to change after arriving home, so I was still sporting a navy blue sleeveless dress that zipped up in the back, with white dog hairs clinging around my hem. We were getting ready to host seventeen adults and eight kids for a big Fourth of July celebration the next day, and I had stock-piled uncooked hamburgers and hot dogs in the refrigerator.

I took the call, then sat down on the steps into the kitchen and hung my head. My mind raced yet seemed blank at the same time. I took the call, then sat down on the steps into the kitchen and hung my head. I tried hard to stifle the flood of emotions, but they still rushed to the surface, a loud cacophony in my head.

Oddly enough, for someone who typically has no problems

sharing her feelings, I had a hard time sorting these out. One of my first thoughts was what a waste it had been, saving all that money for my retirement. I told my husband that since I couldn't take it with me, I needed to go to the mall for a little shopping. Or maybe a lot of shopping. He didn't think that was funny. I thought it was hilarious.

I then went straight to worrying about terrible side effects and how ultimately all this would affect my family. Even though my son was still in high school, the sadness struck me that I might not live to a really ripe old age to be a bother to him and his future family. I'd never felt so vulnerable, so aware that things like this can just *happen*. Which fed into worries about all the what-ifs. I am tough enough to weather a storm, but I'm not so sure about a monsoon, followed by an earthquake, followed by fire from heaven.

We canceled the Fourth of July celebration. We couldn't see past this news to realize that we still had things worth celebrating. I thought of my patients—dogs and cats are so lucky not to have the capacity for worry that we humans (or I) so acutely possess. My dog would have gone ahead with the party with his friends and enjoyed himself—especially with all that ground beef and those hot dogs on offer. Instead, I was left with a bunch of food that I wound up giving away, lest it go to waste. We spent a somber Fourth, when we could have been surrounded by those we love and who love us.

I was anything but joyful as I opened the door to the human

cancer center. My canine patients are typically happy to see the staff as they get to the clinic. They wag their tails in anticipation as they walk through the door, hopeful for a biscuit. No one at the center has ever offered me a piece of Godiva chocolate, although maybe this would be a good trend to start. Frankly, I'm terrified as I head into the elevator and push the button for floor number six. My thoughts are loud, crowding my head. How will I look after going through therapy? What will people think? I know these are superficial concerns, but they still feel crippling. Dogs wear collars, and are put on leashes, but we humans are the ones who feel the restraints of our own insecurities, our own what-ifs, our own doubts about self-worth. But worthiness doesn't have prerequisites.

Fear does not weaken my will; nor my resolve. I hold my head up high and state my name. I am meeting with the medical oncologist to find out what the plan of attack will be. I will gear up for this fight and bring whatever is needed into battle. I am recovering from uterine surgery that I had immediately after my initial diagnosis, and thankfully am healing without complications. I quickly learn that one surgery can cause me to walk like my eighty-one-year-old father, though it took him eighty-one years to develop that slightly bent-over shuffle. Don't get me wrong, I love my dad—I'm just not ready to walk like him.

Unfortunately, despite a favorable pathology report, with a three-millimeter metastatic lesion (spread) in my peritoneum (lower abdomen), my doctor tells me that I will need both chemotherapy and radiation therapy to combat the carcinoma. I have appointments with two other doctors coming up in the next week or so. Until then, I will not have a full plan. The likelihood is that, once I am fully healed from surgery, I will need five and a half weeks of radiation therapy and numerous rounds of chemo. This will run over the course of many months. Turns out I am really, really vain—it upsets me a lot that I will lose my hair.

Dogs and cats don't lose their fur when they receive chemotherapy. That's because, in general, an animal's hair pattern is much different from a human's. Do you ever have to take kitty to the barber because his fur grew too long? No; the majority of animals' fur grows to a certain point and then stops. It sits there in a quiescent stage, whereas our hair grows and grows and grows. Chemotherapy targets the fastest-growing cells; hence our hair is often a goner from treatment. Not so with pets. The exception is dogs that are good for people with allergies, like poodles. Their fur follicles are more like a person's hair in that their fur (or hair) continues to grow, so these kinds of breeds can suffer fur loss.

Losing my hair is nothing compared to the loss of my life, but I bristle at the implications. If I lose my hair, I will look like a C word patient. I never want to show my enemy my weakness, and that includes what grows, or doesn't grow, on my head. When threatened, some dogs can raise their hackles, which makes their hair stand out to give them the appearance of the biggest opponent that they can be. I want to deny that the *C* word has gotten the best of me. I want to be the biggest opponent I can be. But maybe this is like trying to defy gravity. At best, it seems like false bravado.

What floors me is how many random strangers without the *C* word have told me what to do without being asked. It's like when a stranger comes up to a pregnant woman, touches her enlarged belly, and then proceeds to give the mom-to-be unsolicited advice: How to raise the child. What to name the child. I was told that I should just shave my hair in advance, even though it is fine now. First of all, I've never liked being told what to do. Secondly, *really*?! For me, that would be a sign of giving up, and I fight as a matter of principle. I will be the one who goes down with the ship, or at least knows when to man the lifeboats. Perhaps that's a good quality to look for in an oncologist, whether for humans or for animals.

Mrs. Johnson elects the most advanced chemotherapy option for Daisy, and she wants to start right away. Giving me a peek into their family life, she tells me how much they really need the little cocker. She's a vital member of the team, and they love her very much. She provides great joy and is a steadfast companion for Kathy, spending hours by the little girl's side. Kathy is unable to use her hands and arms well enough to dress Daisy—she can't even dress herself—so her parents work as the stylists, decking out Daisy to look like Elsa, Kathy's favorite Disney princess. Kathy relies on her parents—and her dog—to do the many things for herself that we all take for granted. As it turns out, though Daisy has received no formal training whatsoever, she's become a seizure alert therapy dog. Just before Kathy has one of her epileptic episodes, Daisy signals the family so that they can respond accordingly. Ironic as it may be, Daisy has epilepsy herself, though fortunately hers is well controlled with medication. Most important, Daisy doesn't see disability—she sees only Kathy, a loving girl. It doesn't matter that "her" girl can't use words. Daisy knows what Kathy is saying, because she understands her on a deeper level.

As parents, the Johnsons do not know how to broach Daisy's impending mortality with their daughter. Clearly, the prospect weighs heavily on Mrs. Johnson's brow. Talking to a nine-year-old child about their dog's terminal cancer would not be easy for any parent, but for the Johnson family, this has bigger implications. Not only is Daisy a beloved family member, but she's also a necessary part of Kathy's support care.

"Doctor," Mrs. Johnson said, "we really need you to help her live."

Great, I thought. No pressure here.

"We'll do our best," I say, then give the woman a hug. From time to time, we all need a good, long hug.

I take the leash from the woman's hands. Daisy doesn't hesitate. She trots to the back of the hospital with me, curious as to what is around the corner. There will be people back there who will care for her as if she were their own. Cassidy, one of my techs, is quite partial to cocker spaniels, schnauzers, and pit bulls. It's an unusual grouping, but I know that she will love Daisy just a little bit more because of her breed. All my veterinary oncology technicians will carefully administer chemotherapy to help her live and—the big payoff from Daisy's point of view—a treat of a biscuit or two (or three). Daisy clearly loves her treats.

Not surprisingly, Daisy is a very accommodating dog. She readily comes up on the treatment table and allows us to do what we need to do to take care of her. My team flocks around this darling in a blue dress. Cassidy is beside herself with the cocker's cuteness. The professional begins making cooing and baby noises while rubbing behind the spaniel's ears. Daisy presses into her. Clearly, this dog makes friends wherever she goes.

I brief my team about Daisy's cancer and Mrs. Johnson's decision regarding treatment. After weighing the cocker, I calculate her drug dosages and give this information to my head oncology technician, Jackie. I need to decrease Daisy's dose a bit, because some of her weight is due to love handles, rather than muscle mass. Just as in a human hospital, when dealing with chemotherapy, we have to calibrate cautiously for each patient. We also can't risk exposing any employee to chemotherapy, especially when we use it on such a repeated basis.

Jackie makes further calculations, forever meticulous, then begins the process. As will be the case with each chemo treatment, each of us wears a blue chemo-safe gown (aka Smurf-style) over our scrubs, as well as chemo-safe gloves diligently placed over the cuffs of the gown to ensure a tight seal. We also wear safety goggles to protect the eyes and draw up the medication itself in a biologic safety cabinet (think a large, nerdy machine with a big HEPA filter and a fan that exhausts air out through the roof). Jackie puts her long, dark hair up in a ponytail, lest it get in the way of Daisy's chemotherapy.

When I receive my own chemotherapy, I wear my yoga pants (which have never been to yoga) and a zip-up hoodie sweatshirt, not a blue gown like Daisy. I wonder what my doctor would think if I showed up to chemotherapy dressed as Elsa. I never see my treatment team drawing up the drugs, which is done in the hospital's pharmacy. (It's hard to believe they refer to my meds as a "cocktail." "Waiter, any chance I can get a Cosmo instead?") The two nurses on my case come to my hospital room with the chemo drugs, as well as syringes filled with medications to help limit any nausea or allergic reactions. They set these up on the metal stand right next to my bed. It seems like a lot of needles, which is a little intimidating, as is the fact that both nurses are sporting full safety gear. I feel insecure. I've been protecting myself from these scary medications for decades, and yet there I sit, fully exposed, the only one in the room not wearing protection. What's worse, they inject or drip these medications into my vein for hours. Much of this seems to go against the safety precautions I've trained myself to practice. But here I am the patient, not the doctor.

We place Daisy on the treatment table lying down like a sphinx, her forepaws out in front of her. Cassidy gently holds the dog in place while another tech finds a vein on Daisy's right front leg. This isn't easy, with all of her thick, blond fur, but my work team is experienced, and they quickly get a butterfly catheter placed in the vein. Daisy is such a trusting, calm dog—she doesn't even flinch. Cassidy's blond locks rest on Daisy's back as she holds the pet still. I suppose the old adage is correct—some people do look like their favorite dog breeds! Not sure what it says about me, but I like wrinkly, smush-faced dogs and cats.

Daisy receives her chemo through the access port, and within minutes, she's done. She sits up, wagging her tail. She holds no grudges over what just happened. She accepts what has just transpired and is happy to go on with her day. She doesn't look back or worry.

I, on the other hand, agonize about what side effects the chemotherapy has in store for me. I convince myself that if I know what the negative possibilities could be, I can will them away, before they happen. That's a lot of power to presume I have over my outcome, I know. But I imagine I could rise to the occasion.

I bring Daisy back to the waiting room, where Mrs. Johnson and Kathy sit patiently.

"She looks good," the pet parent exclaims. "Did she get her treatment already?"

"Yes, she did great," I assure her. "But we're going to send Daisy home with these two medications, just in case." I hand her a bag with her dog's name on it. "They're to be used if she gets sick—we don't want her to have any side effects. If she has diarrhea or seems nauseated at all, please start the medications right away. Her quality of life is the most important thing. Oh, also, we'll call you tomorrow, to check up on her and see how she's doing."

"Okay, thank you so much," Mrs. Johnson says warmly. We hug again. I can feel the woman's shoulders drop, as if her entire body took a deep sigh.

"Can I help you to your car?" I offer. This mom needs a third arm.

"No, I'm good. Thank you, though," she says, as she navigates Kathy's wheelchair while holding on to Daisy's leash, her X-rays, and the bag of medications.

The following day, I call Mrs. Johnson to ask how Daisy's doing after her chemotherapy.

"She actually seems better than before. Is it possible she would have *more* energy after treatment?"

"You know, a lot of people ask that. Many dogs do seem to feel better on chemotherapy. I think we don't realize that the cancer causes a pet to be quieter at home, competing with some of its energy. Some people chalk it up to arthritis or age, and then once their dog receives chemotherapy, they realize it was the cancer causing the lethargy. Either way, I'm so glad she's feeling good."

Mrs. Johnson pauses, then asks, "Why did Daisy get the cancer? Should I have done something differently?" I can hear the guilt in her voice. So many times, I am asked about the water a pet drinks, the food they eat, chemicals spread on the lawn. And the list goes on . . .

"You didn't cause Daisy's cancer," I begin. "Cancer in pets, just like in people, can happen for a multitude of reasons. Some cancers are more prevalent in certain breeds because they're passed down genetically. Some cancers have a higher rate of occurrence for pets that live in households in which family members smoke. Some cancers can be caused from the sun. There is even one cancer in dogs that can be spread through sex! In cats, one-third of all those afflicted with feline leukemia virus (a poor name, because it's not really leukemia at all), will eventually develop cancer from that virus."

"So, I didn't *cause* this to happen to Daisy?"

"Not at all. Lymphoma is often, though not always, genetically spread, and the genetics of it tend to go back many, many decades. Even so, animals have been getting cancer since the beginning of time. We have proof that even dinosaurs developed some malignant forms of cancer, such as bone cancer and leukemia. You take very good care of Daisy. You feed her a high-quality food and give her lots of love."

"Well, she takes good care of us. Oh, and I forgot to ask, will she lose her fur?"

"No, she shouldn't. Cats don't lose their fur on chemotherapy, and the majority of dogs don't either. It's because Daisy's fur is different from a person's hair."

"That's interesting," she said. "But we'd love her just the same if she were as bald as a cue ball." And with that, we hung up.

A week goes by, and Daisy returns for her recheck appointment. Once again, Mrs. Johnson is accompanied by Kathy, seated in her wheelchair. I greet them both in the waiting room. Bending down next to Kathy, I ask her how her day is and how her dog is doing. If she was shy at the initial consultation for Daisy, today she is very eager to interact with me. I tell her how good Daisy looks in Elsa's dress, and that she has good taste. It's clear she understands what I'm saying, and she shows her delight with a beaming smile. I then look up at Mrs. Johnson, who asks how I am.

"I'm fine, thank you. More importantly, how's Daisy?"

She gives me her own warm smile as she pushes back a strand of dark hair from her daughter's face.

"If we didn't know it, it's as if nothing is wrong with her. Is that normal?"

"That's how it's supposed to be. I'm so glad! If it's okay with you, I'm going to take Daisy to the back for some blood work, and then I'll do a physical exam on her."

"She'll follow you anywhere as long as you have biscuits," Mrs. Johnson says with a wink.

She hands me the dog's leash, then I wave at Kathy, who throws me another smile that lights up the waiting room. Daisy trots alongside me, through the door and into the oncology treatment area.

I lower the exam table and the cocker hops on top. I raise the table while Daisy sits there calmly. Cassidy is eager to see her new friend. After my team draws her blood to check her white blood cell count, I feel under the dog's neck. These lymph nodes are normal. I check her prescapular, or shoulder, lymph nodes. Normal as well. Both her axillary and groin lymph nodes are just fine. And her popliteal lymph nodes, the nodes behind her knee region, have gone back to normal size as well.

I suspect that the Johnsons could really use positive news, and I look forward to telling them Daisy's results. After reviewing her blood work, I head back to the waiting room while my team treats the canine with her next chemotherapy drug. With a big smile on my face, I tell Mrs. Johnson the wonderful news, and a tear falls down her cheek. Kathy watches her mom quickly brush it away, and I give the woman another hug, a happy embrace. My technician brings Daisy up to us, and I remind the pet parent that we need to see the dog back in one week.

Mrs. Johnson diligently returns as scheduled, and each week the dog comes dressed as a Disney princess: Belle, Cinderella, Snow White. But just like Kathy, I think the best is Daisy as Elsa. Girlfriend looks good in blue. Many times, Mrs. Johnson brings Daisy in alone. Occasionally, Kathy will be at her side.

One day, on a routine chemotherapy visit, Mrs. Johnson arrives with a worried look on her face. In her wheelchair, Kathy seems unusually subdued. The mother tells my technician that she noticed some lumps on Daisy and thinks the cancer has returned. There is no princess dress on the dog, no radiant smile on Kathy's face. My tech, Cassidy, is concerned as well, and brings the canine to the back for me to examine. With the cocker atop the exam table, I feel her lymph nodes—in her neck, in her shoulders, the axilla and groin regions, and behind her knees. I palpate them all a second time, wanting to be sure. They are all fine. Daisy continues to be in a remission. She does have two new soft tissue masses on the top of her back, but in no way are these related to her lymphoma.

"You're such a good girl!'" Cassidy exclaims, happy for the good news. The technician then holds the dog still as I take samples from both masses with a needle and syringe. Under the microscope, it is evident that these are lipomas, or benign fatty cysts. As an older cocker spaniel, Daisy has numerous warts and sebaceous cysts on her body. While her blood work is being processed, I head to the waiting room to alleviate Mrs. Johnson's fears.

"How is she, Doc?" she asks, rising quickly from her chair. Her blue eyes eagerly scan my face.

"Daisy's just fine. Those lumps you noticed are benign lipomas. They have nothing to do with her cancer. She'll likely get more of these fatty masses as she gets older. Just like the cysts she already has."

I watch as relief sweeps over Mrs. Johnson's face. I bend down and put my hand on top of Kathy's leg. Kathy understands that the news is good. An ear-to-ear grin lights up her face.

"We say those are her old lady warts," Mrs. Johnson says with a chuckle. "But we love her, warts and all. In our house, we've learned to celebrate all of our imperfections. And Daisy certainly has plenty to celebrate, doesn't she, Kathy?"

She says this with a bit of a giggle, then gives me a hug of gratitude. I turn to go to the back to check on the cocker's blood work and approve her chemotherapy dose.

Mrs. Johnson has given me something to think about. If only we all felt free enough to celebrate our imperfections, life might be a little less grim, a bit more joyful. I say that as my hair grows thinner on top of my head. I have officially set the steps in place for a *w-i-g*. I prefer not to say the word, but I want to be ahead of this concern, so I consider my options. I have also considered self-induced "house arrest," just staying home until everything grows back. However, regrowth may take more time than I could stand to hide out. But there's a confounding issue. I feel like a fake in a *w-i-g*, and I have never been fake. I can't even do fake nails. Not even when Lee Press-On Nails were all the rage. I feel like a wig or a hat would be me hiding behind a costume. I want to be me, warts and all.

As another option, I heard something about a type of cooling cap that can be worn on a person's head to try to save one's follicles. I will investigate this further to see if it is a decent option for me. I know my hair obsession isn't rational. If it were a girlfriend of mine or even sweet Daisy, I would not look at them any differently whether they had hair (or fur) or not. And I do know that my friends would feel the same

26

about me. But I would feel as if everyone were feeling sorrow, or pity. Deep down, I don't want to seem "different," or simply without hair (can't say the word "bald"), for Peter, my dear son. I am supposed to be strong for him. I don't want him to feel bad or pity me. I guess I've chosen the right profession. A running joke among veterinarians is that our patients don't care what we look like, what we're wearing, or whether we've combed whatever hair we have or don't have. Throw in a pass for not brushing your teeth, and this might be a good job for a middle school boy.

Five months pass, and thankfully Daisy continues to do well. Her warts grow a bit, but no one notices when she sports her princess outfit. Mrs. Johnson is a master at balancing her home responsibilities with bringing their cocker spaniel in for treatment. I am in awe at how she handles it with such a sweet, peaceful outlook.

But one day, the Johnsons don't show up for Daisy's routine recheck chemo appointment. The receptionist calls the family in an attempt to reschedule, but she is limited to leaving a message on their voice mail. At first, I don't think anything of it—everyone forgets things at some point. The following day, however, the Johnsons have not returned our call. Something is not right. Days go by and still there's no word from the family. Despite a few more calls made on our end, I do not hear from Mrs. Johnson until a full two weeks have gone by.

"Line one, Mrs. Johnson with Daisy, line one," blares over the intercom. I rush to the phone.

"Hi, how are you?" I ask in a hurried tone. There is a deep sigh on the other end of the receiver.

"We've had a bit of a doozy these couple of weeks," Mrs. Johnson offers. "I'm so sorry that we missed Daisy's appointment."

"It's no problem at all. Is everything okay? We've been concerned."

"Kathy had a bit of a setback. It started with what we thought was a cold, but because she's so sedentary, the infection quickly moved into her lungs. We've gone through this before," the mother confides. "She couldn't breathe. We ended up having to take her out of state by ambulance, on oxygen, to the children's hospital that has helped her with other medical problems. Kathy was in the ICU for ten days."

"I am so sorry. How is she now?" I ask cautiously.

"Oh, she's better. We're home. We still have to do nebulization treatments on her, but she's better." I can hear the exhaustion in Mrs. Johnson's voice.

"I'm so glad she's better. You're an amazing mom and a very strong woman. Your family is fortunate to have you." With that, I book Daisy an appointment for the next day and hang up.

I sit down, a bit shaken. I cannot imagine the worry that likely filled the family. And their incredible fortitude! It will be nice to see Mrs. Johnson and her dog. Thankfully, Daisy has been doing so well, the missed weeks should not be too much of a strain with her cancer.

Since my own diagnosis, everyone I interact with tells me how strong I am, that they'd crumble if they were in my shoes. Is that what someone should say to a person going through this, I wonder, that they're strong? Is a person born inherently strong, or is it that circumstances condition us to be so? Aren't we all strong when we need to be, when life dishes out the really tough stuff? Compared to all that the Johnson family has to deal with, though, my problems are small potatoes.

Daisy returns the next day. At the "owner" end of her bright pink leash is Mrs. Johnson, worn out. The oncology nurse greets the duo happily. Kathy has been left at home while recovering. The technician brings the dog back and places her on the exam table. While holding my breath, I do a physical on Daisy. "Thank goodness," I say out loud. Then I breathe normally again. Daisy's exam is just fine. The cocker has her routine blood work performed and receives her chemotherapy (and her cookie) without incident.

Over the next year, Kathy has two more hospitalization episodes. They're always scary, yet Mrs. Johnson continues to balance the care of her daughter with her dedication to Daisy. Two more years pass, and thankfully, Daisy miraculously continues to stay in a remission. Clearly, our "Elsa" has not read the rule book on her disease. By year three, we see the Johnsons only periodically.

Daisy is now a fourteen-year-old dog. Through all the years I've taken care of her, she's never missed a beat. Through the many appointments, I have seen the family's unending love for Kathy, and I have learned about the kindness and gentleness they all express on a daily basis. I used to say that the Johnsons have earned their spot in heaven with their care of Kathy, and with their devotion to Daisy. As far as I'm concerned, they could rob a bank and still go right through those pearly gates. But being able to help their dog in this small way, and to learn from their example, I am the one who is blessed.

2

BENTLEY

H ey, Doc, who's gonna die first?"

I did a double take, my mind racing. "Excuse me?"

Is this man sitting across from me trying to be funny? Or difficult?

"No really, Doc, who's gonna die first?"

This is my 1:00 p.m. appointment; it's a day like any other. Except this is a new patient. Mr. Bean and his dog have come to see me about a biopsy that their veterinarian did last week. Bentley is a low-to-the-ground, overweight tricolor beagle, a neutered male nine years of age. He looks at me, panting, the dog's belly barely above the beige linoleum floor. His red nylon leash leads up to a gentleman most likely in his early sixties. Mr. Bean is dressed in a brown suit, complete with a tweed vest. He seems nervous, on edge, which is understandable when one needs to see any oncologist, whether in veterinary or human medicine. His foot is tapping with displaced energy.

I begin with my routine set of questions to better understand Bentley's case. "Has he had any past medical issues? How long has he strained to urinate? Have you noticed any blood in his urine?" Mr. Bean responds in short, curt answers. It is clear that either he does not want to be at this appointment, or he got up on the wrong side of the bed this morning. Or maybe every morning. But getting a good history makes for better care of the patient, and so I persist.

"How is Bentley's appetite? Has he lost any weight?"

"He's a beagle, for heaven's sake! Of course he has a good appetite. Does he look like he's lost any weight?"

I offer a faint smile. The man just glares back at me, his arms crossed. I lift Bentley onto the exam table and let out a little groan. I won't need to work out today. I begin my physical examination—looking in his mouth, at his ears and eyes, listening to his chest, feeling his abdomen.

"Would you mind if I did a rectal exam on Bentley?" I ask Mr. Bean.

"I assumed you would. Do whatever you need to," he replies while turning slightly away.

I ask one of my oncology nurses to come into the exam room to hold Bentley for me. No one likes having a rectal done, and the flip side of that same coin is that no one really likes to do it. But it's part of the job, and a whole lot better than when I was in veterinary school. For cow evaluations, our rectal "glove" was a long rubber sleeve that went all the way up to my shoulder for sanitary protection. Not the latest in fashion but highly recommended for the business at hand.

I put on an exam glove and add a bit of K-Y Jelly for lubrication to ease insertion. The technician holds Bentley, and he's a good boy and doesn't squirm. I put my index finger in, and I can feel his prostate gland. In a neutered male dog, I should not be able to feel this organ at all unless there's an infection, or a cyst, or cancer. Sadly, Bentley's prostate is three centimeters in size, as big as an unshelled walnut. Additionally, Bentley's enlarged prostate is irregular in shape and pushing up on his colon, or large intestine. This can make it more difficult for feces to pass through.

"Does Bentley strain at all when he is defecating?" I ask the man.

"No, not really," Mr. Bean says.

"Are his stools ever thinner, smaller, or ribbon-like in shape?"

"Well, now that you mention it, I suppose they are a bit thinner."

Bentley has prostatic carcinoma—cancer of the prostate gland. It is not a terribly common disease in dogs, though it can occur in males as they get older. Cats don't have to worry about this cancer because they don't have prostate glands.

Sometimes in dogs, the condition can be more aggressive than it is in people. In part, this may be due to its being a more virulent disease in animals, or it could be because we diagnose it later in dogs, who can't tell us that something's not right. I suggest to Mr. Bean that a stool softener would help his dog.

Bentley's stools are thinner because his enlarged prostate is pushing up on his intestine, narrowing the lumen, making it more difficult for feces to pass. Though Metamucil works, pets don't like it. Fortunately, canned pumpkin can be a good alternative. Typically, dogs eat it readily. As a beagle, and thus always ready to eat, Bentley should have no trouble getting it down.

At the time I was treating Bentley, our only real option for prostate cancer was chemotherapy. Nowadays, we know that this disease can also respond well to radiation. Mr. Bean listens impatiently as I describe the various chemotherapy options.

Pets do remarkably well with treatment. Your next-door neighbor's dog could have been on chemotherapy though you might never have noticed. While some cats and dogs can have vomiting or diarrhea, it's uncommon. In part, this is due to the fact that their veterinary oncologists give them lower doses of medications than their human counterparts receive, the reason being that we're striving more for quality of life, while extending it for a longer time, versus a cure.

Even though Mr. Bean looks bored, we go over side effects and costs. Fortunately for Bentley, there is only a 15 percent chance that he will get sick with this treatment. He may turn down food for a few days or have some stomach upset. Mr. Bean lets out a very loud huff, but I continue on. There is also a chance, albeit quite small, that Bentley's heart could be affected. The chemotherapy drug can cause damage to the cardiac muscle and can even cause heart failure. We should check Bentley's heart first, to make sure that we're starting with no structural issues. Mr. Bean says he has no further questions and tells me that he needs to get on with his day. It turns out that "Mr. Bean" is actually "Dr. Bean," a psychiatrist.

Despite his seeming detachment, Dr. Bean elects to begin chemotherapy. He wants to do anything necessary to help his four-legged companion. Bentley begins to vocalize, braying as only a hound can do. I offer him some biscuits and he gobbles them down. (He knows how to work the room.) Bentley's treatment schedule will be such that I see him once every three weeks for intravenous chemotherapy for a total of five treatments. Bentley's appointments will be no more than thirty minutes long, but it is clear from his scowl and tapping foot that Dr. Bean would rather be anyplace but here. Bentley follows me into the back, nose to the ground, discovering new smells along the way.

My oncology team of three greets Bentley with open arms.

He wags his tail, and they give him a few more snacks. Some would call those bribes—Bentley just sees them as delicious. Either way, they do the trick. He feels comfortable with the team right away. They take Bentley down the hall for an ultrasound of his heart. It is a nice feature of working in a large veterinary hospital, having various specialists who are able to collaborate, bringing a pet the best possible care. I watch as his nose leads the way.

Bentley lies on his side on the table, while a technician shaves a small patch of fur where the transducer will be placed, so that our cardiologist can perform the ultrasound, or echocardiogram. The vet measures the size of each of the four chambers in Bentley's heart, then assesses blood flow and takes further measurements. When I check in, the cardiologist tells me that the beagle's heart is just fine, good to go for chemotherapy.

I walk Bentley back to my area, where two technicians do an ECG of his heart to give us a baseline recording. Having this pre-treatment reading, we can compare this with future ECGs to make sure that we are doing no harm. We want to do our best to protect this vital organ.

While my technician, Jackie, begins to draw up the chemotherapy drugs, I go out to the waiting room to inform Dr. Bean of the echocardiogram results. He greets me with a blank stare.

"Okay, well, we will start his first chemo now," I say gently while walking backward to the treatment area, still facing Dr. Bean. The man's face doesn't change.

Bentley is once again lying on his side on the treatment table when I walk into the room. Two technicians are holding him as Jackie places Bentley's catheter in his right hind leg vein—success on the first try. This isn't her first rodeo. Each tech is wearing her protective gear.

I tell my team of my difficulty connecting with Dr. Bean, the obstacle of his cold manner.

"He'd better be nice to you," Jackie inserts. "I mean it."

Forever the protector, Jackie is always on guard for my well-being, as well as the well-being of her coworkers. Standing at five foot eight, she takes guff from no one.

"He's fine, really," I assure her. "Something just seems off. I wouldn't expect someone who listens for a living to be like this."

Over the course of ten minutes, the red liquid is slowly administered into Bentley's vein while he lies there quietly, listening to the "Good boy" and "Good dog" praise offered to keep him calm and unstressed. Ten minutes, though, can seem so much longer. Once the syringe is empty, the techs remove his catheter, then place a bandage over the site for pressure to stop any bleeding. Bentley receives a few more biscuits, then we escort him back to his "dad." The gentleman reaches for the leash, turns to walk away, and mumbles a barely audible, "Thank you."

I call Dr. Bean the next day, to see how Bentley is doing after his first treatment. There is no answer. I leave a message but it is never returned.

Three weeks later, the beagle comes sniffing through the door for his recheck appointment, right on time. Jackie takes a brief history from Dr. Bean.

"He seems a little quieter lately," the doctor expresses. "He's been sleeping a lot and doesn't bark at the mail carrier anymore. He's still eating like a Hoover vacuum, though."

The technician tells Dr. Bean that she will take Bentley to the back for his blood work, after which the vet will be out to talk with him. When I see Bentley, I notice that he seems sluggish. He still pines for a biscuit, but he is not his inquisitive self. I do a physical exam while the lab test is running, and though his evaluation is unremarkable, it's clear there is something wrong. I hear the beep, beep, beep of the machine as my team performs an ECG. Thankfully, this is not the cause of his lethargy. Just then, I receive Bentley's blood work, hot off the press. Bentley has a low white blood cell count. We need our white blood cells to fight off infection. Our body makes these very fast-growing cells in our bone marrow, and chemotherapy often targets the fastest-

growing cells. I ask the technician to take Bentley's temperature. It's 103.8 degrees Fahrenheit. While this is high, it is
not dangerously high for a dog. Cats and dogs have a higher
body temperature than we do. Typically, from 100 up to
102.5 degrees Fahrenheit is considered normal. But 103.8,
in an unstressed dog, especially coupled with a low white
blood cell count, is concerning.

I remember back to how I felt after one of my own chemotherapy treatments. I had gone to the hospital two weeks
afterward and was not feeling well at all—no energy whatsoever. The phlebotomist took a blood sample. Turns out, my
neutrophil count (the specific white blood cells that fight off
infection) was extremely low. Normal is a minimum of 1,600
cells or more, though ideally, you'd have 3,000 or more. Mine
was 100! This is where a little bit of knowledge can be a very
bad thing, and I got really scared. I understood the risks, and
I knew the worst-case scenarios. With such a low count, I was
more susceptible to getting an infection from what might
barely make another person sneeze. And I knew that there
was a small chance, thankfully quite small, of not being able
to come back from such a low number. Yep, not good to know.

The ER doctor started me on oral antibiotics to guard
against infection and also gave me an injection to help my
bone marrow make new white cells. I made sure that I iso-
lated in the house to limit my contact with germs. The next
day I got another blood test to evaluate my count. Luckily for

me, I started willing up my cells while I was still at the hospital. Don't laugh; I'm convinced it worked. Of course, this was after three days of injections, three visits to the hospital, and a full week of antibiotics. But I willed them up, just the same.

Bentley is sent home on oral antibiotics to help guard against infection. Given how much the dog loves his groceries, it will be very easy for Dr. Bean to give him his medication twice a day for seven days. We postpone Bentley's chemotherapy by one week. If we simply continued his treatment, we would make his cells go down even lower, which could be quite dangerous. Dr. Bean doesn't even look at us as we discharge Bentley. He quickly scrambles out the door.

Bentley returns the following week, punctual as usual, and evidently feeling much better. Pulling at the end of his leash, his nose guiding him on a new scent, he no longer shows any signs of lethargy. Cassidy takes the beagle to the back to check his blood count. I perform a physical exam and this time repeat a rectal exam as well. He stands like a trooper. Though I can still feel Bentley's prostate gland, it has reduced in size to 2.25 centimeters—down three-quarters of a centimeter. Not bad for just one dose of chemotherapy. My technician returns with the dog's blood work results. Fortunately, his white count is now normal. I discuss both of these good findings with Dr. Bean, yet he displays no emotion when I relay the happy news. I go over the plan once more, saying that we will reduce Bentley's dose a bit with the hope that his white cell count does not drop down into a dangerous level again. Dr. Bean nods in agreement but says not a word. I look at the psychiatrist for a few seconds, then turn on my heel to take care of Bentley. The treatment is uneventful, and Dr. Bean hurries out with his dog.

On Bentley's fourth visit, I walk out to the pair and sit down next to Dr. Bean in the waiting room. He taps his right foot. He looks at me, and I look back. Healing and caring for someone, even a furry four-legged someone, requires understanding and compassion among everyone involved. I extend an olive branch. "How are you today, Dr. Bean?"

"You know, you never answered my question."

"Which question was that?"

"Which one of us will die first, me or him?"

I search his face, trying to uncover why he is asking me this. I have certainly had clients who were quite old, caring for a young dog, wondering if they will be able to keep up with an energetic pup. That concern is obvious. This is not so apparent. Dr. Bean is in his early sixties. For all intents and purposes, he seems healthy to me. Of course, I thought I was healthy, and then I was told I had the *C* word, so what do I know?

Dr. Bean begins to talk. It is as if through all of Bentley's appointments, he has kept everything bottled up. And today, finally, he is uncorked. As he shares, Dr. Bean's face begins to soften, he relaxes, and his shoulders settle downward.

He tells me that he loves being a psychiatrist, and that he believes in the good work of the medical profession. One year ago, Dr. Bean began having GI issues. A little diarrhea here, a little temporary bloating there. But as the weeks turned into months, his clinical signs progressed, and his GI issues made it difficult for him to go about his standard day. Dr. Bean saw an internist who scheduled him for a colonoscopy with a gastrointestinal specialist. He complied with the unpleasant preparation period that no one likes: not eating anything the night before, drinking what seems like an endless supply of a terrible liquid, and the numerous bathroom trips. The results of the colonoscopy came back nonspecific—nothing to be concerned about. However, Dr. Bean's symptoms grew worse. Rounds of different medications would show promise, but then his symptoms would return in full force. Finally, months later, he underwent a repeat colonoscopy, and then more tests.

"I have advanced-stage colon cancer," Dr. Bean confides. My heart sinks. I put my hand on his arm.

Dr. Bean stares down at the ground, Bentley whimpering by his side. "I don't have long to live," he admits.

Suddenly it all makes sense. How difficult it must be for him, knowing that he and his dog are both running out of time. And here is this person I thought I knew, who appeared so irritated with Bentley's chemotherapy appointments, who was really irritated with life in general. Dr. Bean tells me that through everything that he's had to endure, the various chemotherapy protocols, the radiation therapy treatments, the experimental medications, Bentley has never left his side. When Dr. Bean could only lie in bed, recovering from a procedure he hoped would slow his cancer, Bentley would lie there with him. Bentley didn't ask to play ball or to go outside on long walks. He didn't bark or bray; he just stayed at his pet parent's side, letting him get much-needed rest.

Conversely, when Dr. Bean was having a good day, Bentley was there again, eager to accompany his owner, tail wagging, happy to enjoy the time that was ahead. Bentley lived in the moment, accepting each day for what it was. And now this man wants to do everything he can for his steadfast companion. Dr. Bean wants to be the pillar of strength for his dog that his dog has been for him. As hard as it's been for Dr. Bean to come into this veterinary hospital, being reminded of what he himself is going through, Bentley always seems happy to see us. Dr. Bean wants to give Bentley quality time for however long he can. Bentley fights his diagnosis not with stoic bravery, but by taking each moment as it comes, enjoying what's in front of him. But clearly and understandably, this is not easy for Dr. Bean.

Overriding all this is Dr. Bean's desperate fear of leaving Bentley behind. And yet the good doctor is torn over the potential of having to grieve the loss of Bentley should Bentley pass away first.

"So, who is going to die first? Me or him?" he asks me again.

How can I answer this? They are in a race against time, a race that neither wants to finish. It doesn't seem fair. At least that's what my medical team always told me: cancer isn't fair. But that's no comfort at this time. I'm not sure it's ever comforting. It may be true, but it's not what you want to hear.

"I, I don't know," I stammer back, in a barely audible voice. Isn't that great, years of being a veterinarian and that's the first thing out of my mouth? Dr. Bean is still looking at me.

"I don't know," I repeat, perhaps a little more convincingly this time. "But I do know that you are here now. And you are here to help Bentley. And Bentley is as happy as he can be. Thankfully, your dog has not experienced many side effects. Furthermore, he should continue to do well with the remainder of his treatments. And you've given him more happy days. It's so hard for all of us to be in the moment, but Bentley is doing just that. He's happy that the sun comes up each day. He's excited for each silly dog biscuit that he gets. And he loves being with you. Most important, you have this time together."

I realized early on that for me, a huge silver lining in the diagnosis I'd fought with conviction was that I had so many amazing people in my life. I think I'd lost myself a bit over the past year or so before this all happened. I'd been working a tremendous amount, keeping my head above water as a veterinarian, a mom, a wife, and with life in general, but I was running myself ragged. And I felt lonely. Looking back, I wouldn't have changed any of my choices, but this diagnosis has given me pause, given me the time to come back to me. I learned (damn hard lesson) that I was not, am not, alone. And I cherished the time that my friends and family spent with me, driving me to treatments, bringing me comforts when I was not feeling well.

I am slowly learning the sanctity of self-care. I'm better at taking care of others than taking care of myself, but I'm trying to learn. My self-esteem used to come from checking items off of my "To Do" list each day. I have yet to find the joy in being good to myself, but I have put some things in place. I know it's important to give back to myself so I can be filled up, and so I can keep on giving. If we don't fill up, we'll have nothing left to give. This is a lesson I learned too late, but that I am desperate to mirror for my teenage son, so that he doesn't run himself down to the bone, always put himself last. I'm not saying that had I done things differently, I wouldn't have gotten that *C* word diagnosis. But I am saying that I sure could have been a lot more loving to myself in the past, and still can today. Life is always a work in progress, and I have a long way to go. But I'm more aware, and I'm trying to be kinder to myself. I will try to eat well and rest and listen carefully to my body, which hadn't been heard in a while. Actually, I did hear it, but I plowed ahead anyway.

I don't know that there was any one particular symptom that I ignored. Rather, it was a whole mess of symptoms, of my body telling me that it was at its limit. I was terribly exhausted, burning the candle at both ends. I would fall asleep the moment I sat down on the sofa in the early evening. And yet, I would wake up at two in the morning, my head aflutter with all of life's issues. Makeup couldn't fully cover the dark circles beneath my eyes. My eczema was in full force (of course only on my face)—but it always comes out to party when I am overly stressed. On top of all of this, I just didn't feel great. But I pressed on anyway. I convinced myself that taking care of everything else was more important than adding myself to the list of things that needed care.

I lead Bentley to the back. We take his blood to check his counts. Fortunately, the chemotherapy dose reduction did the trick: Bentley has a normal white blood cell level, so it will be safe for him to receive his third treatment. His ECG and physical exam are unremarkable. Bentley then assumes the position for his rectal exam—I think he'd do anything for the promise of a biscuit. The beagle's mass has shrunk one centimeter, bringing his prostate to 1.25 centimeters, barely palpable. Bentley lies on his side for the chemotherapy to be injected into his left hind leg. My team is careful with the drug administration. All the while, I'm still pondering Dr. Bean's question.

Three weeks to the day later, Bentley arrives in the waiting room for his recheck appointment. Though my team and I are still in the back, we can hear his beagle bark. Time to get Bentley!

The dog is doing well, Dr. Bean tells Jackie, who now has a soft spot in her heart for this man. Bentley is eager to go to the back, pulling on the leash—he knows where we keep the treats. After doing the physical exam, rectal, ECG, and reviewing Bentley's blood work, I head up front to talk with Dr. Bean. He's seated in a bank of open chairs, almost smiling, and is no longer wearing the three-piece suit. Today, he is in a pair of khakis and a navy fleece jacket. There is no foot tapping, no scowl on his face. He seems almost the slightest bit happy to be here. I sit down next to him.

"How are you today?" I ask.

"How's Bentley?"

"Bentley is doing well. His physical exam is fine, his blood work is normal, and I can no longer feel an enlarged prostate on him. Oh, and he's gained weight. How are you?" I ask again.

Dr. Bean smiles a smile of relief. "I'm doing okay. Some days are better than others, but today is a good day. So, my dog is okay?"

"Yes, he's good," I reassure him. I notice that Dr. Bean looks a bit paler than when we first met two months ago; he appears a bit thinner as well. I ask if he's able to work as much and how that's going, which prompts him to tell me about his practice, and how he is fortunate despite his health. The psychiatrist is able to sit with his patients, listen, and provide guidance. He shares with me how there are so many people he treats who struggle with addiction, and how pervasive this is in our society. The epidemic perplexes him, yet he is dedicated to helping where he can.

While we sit and chat, the oncology team diligently gives Bentley his intravenous chemotherapy. They bring him up front, which ends my conversation with Dr. Bean.

"Until next time," I say fondly.

"Until next time," he says back. I detect a note of kindness in his voice.

I "see" people's scars every day at work with clients, in my family, with my dear friends. Dr. Bean certainly has more than his fair share. I, personally, am accumulating more scars than I ever wanted. Sure, I have scars on my abdomen from my surgery, the bandages covering them, as if I'd forget. But these scars are expected and can be addressed with ointments and antibiotics. The other, developing scars I have from this are so much deeper and harder to soothe. Scars affect how we act and how we respond to whatever comes our way. Some of us hide our scars; others wear them on their sleeves. It is my goal in veterinary medicine to help pet parents through a tough time, to minimize any new scar formation, and to offer knowledge and compassion when the world can seem so cruel. A hand on one's shoulder or a sincere hug can be the best non-medicine around.

It is a busy three weeks with new clients calling, trying to be fit in to see us when an appointment slot doesn't exist. Cancer doesn't have a busy season, but lately, for whatever reason, it seems as if new cases are coming out of the wood-work. It's hard to turn away new patients, especially when they're all facing cancer in one form or another. The pet parents are worried, wanting to understand their pet's disease.

I don't notice that Dr. Bean has postponed Bentley's final appointment until the following week. When Dr. Bean and Bentley do arrive, they're punctual as usual—simply one week late.

"Hey, Bentley boy, how ya doing?" Jackie asks as the beagle looks up at her, tail wagging, his tongue hanging out as he pants. Dr. Bean comments that the dog is well, no problems to report. Bentley trots to the back, ready to give a blood sample in exchange for a few Milk Bones. I perform the customary physical exam and rectal exam and evaluate his ECG. Thankfully, I will have only good news to report to Bentley's dad today. I know this will make him happy.

I head out the door to the waiting room but slow my gait as I see Dr. Bean, sitting a bit slumped, not looking as dapper as usual, his face slightly drawn. He's wearing his blue fleece, but this time with gray sweatpants instead of khakis. On seeing me, though, he sits up and smiles. He tries to hide how bad he's feeling.

"Hi, how are you today?" I ask quietly as I sit down next to him.

"I'm doing okay," he offers. "This is one of those not-good days. But I'll be fine. How's my Bentley?"

"Bentley is doing well. Everything's normal. And the best news is, today is his last treatment!" I smile a big smile. "We should see Bentley back in a couple of months, just to check him out and make sure he's continuing to do well. At that time, we might do an abdominal ultrasound to further assess his belly." Dr. Bean nods in agreement.

"You know what's hard?" Dr. Bean confides. "That my mom has to see her son face his own mortality. It's not supposed to be like this," he adds.

He's right. The pain and sadness that she feels evidently weigh heavily on her son.

"I wish it didn't have to be this way," he says.

I ask Dr. Bean if I can give him a hug, and he accepts.

We hug for a moment, and as he starts to let go, I hold on. Sometimes, you just need a real hug when life is awfully hard, and I know that this man, however formal and reserved, is no different. I feel his shoulders drop, and I feel him relax. When he sighs, tears well up in my eyes.

We let go of the embrace just as Bentley comes bounding through the door, two technicians at his heels. I quickly wipe the moisture from my eyes. The dog barks and we all chuckle. Jackie, Cassidy, and I watch as Dr. Bean and Bentley walk slowly toward the door. Bentley always takes his cue from his two-legged family member.

I never heard back from Dr. Bean once Bentley was done with his chemotherapy. I realized how much I'd looked forward to each of their visits, and I wished we'd talked more than we did.

In the veterinary world, in general, no news is good news, but in this case, I always wondered what happened. A year later, I tried to find Dr. Bean online. Sadly, he'd passed away, but the tributes so many of his patients gave him were nothing short of amazing. They thanked Dr. Bean for improving their lives; in some cases, saving their lives. I was blessed to know Dr. Bean as well as his friend Bentley, and to witness how much they helped each other. I never did find out what happened at the end of the race. I still don't want to know. I like to imagine that Bentley and Dr. Bean are together again, happy.

3

COSMO

I start appointments early each day, preferring not to have anything hanging over my head. I'd rather roll up the proverbial sleeves and get crackin'.

In my veterinary practice, during these early hours, the waiting room is empty, and the phones are quiet. It's a nice time to arrive—peaceful and calm.

When I go in for my own RT treatments, if I've scheduled one of the cancer center's first morning appointment slots, it's the exact opposite. The hospital is bustling with activity. A bunch of us are sitting there, waiting for the radiation team to begin their day. Whenever someone checks in at the reception desk, he or she has to give their name and birth date. It feels like name, rank, and serial number. And none of these soldiers volunteered.

We sit in silence, looking down at our phones, each of us wanting to get it over with and get out of there as quickly as possible. Some individuals are headed for work; some will head back home and pile into bed. We all seem, or at least I certainly feel, a bit nervous. In general, no one speaks, but we all know what each of us is going through. Even so, I can't help wanting to connect with anyone who sits next to me or even reasonably nearby. "So, what are you in for?" I sometimes ask, as if the diagnosis were a jail sentence, and we're heading for the slammer. I actually think I'm kind of funny, but I don't think my "cellmates" always see the humor.

It's not easy to have to have radiation therapy every single day. However, I am very lucky that each time I arrive at the center, I'm never alone. My loving husband or one of my dear friends insists on accompanying me. Still, I've met a few ladies with whom I've developed an ongoing waiting-room relationship. I look for them each time I come, hoping to see a familiar face and to hear how they're doing. Each of these waiting-room buddies comes alone. Janice, in for breast cancer, is from the Upper East Side of Manhattan. We always chat just a bit, encouraging each other while trying to fill the void before our names are called for treatment. It's odd which part of the "necessary losses" each of us struggles with. Janice's biggest fear, from receiving chemotherapy and radiation therapy, is losing her eyelashes. Mine have already jumped ship. We refer to her lashes as her "little friends." The fact that she's lost her hair doesn't seem to bother her so much, maybe because she looks quite good in her wig.

A woman from Newark is actually glad about her hair loss, because she's always struggled with dreaded facial hair, and now that's no longer an issue. Another woman had shaved her head from time to time as a fashion statement, so hair loss doesn't faze her. A fourth woman doesn't care if she only has a few strands; she isn't going to let any of them go. For me, I mourn the loss of each and every follicle.

Back at work, I enter the exam room to meet my first appointment of the day. Cosmo Engel is a neutered, fourteen-year-old, eighty-seven-pound golden retriever. In reviewing his medical record prior to this appointment, I discovered that he'd had an enormous number of medical problems in the past: ongoing thyroid disease, three other cancers that he's beat, arthritis, knee surgery, laryngeal paralysis, a history of aspiration pneumonia, and heart disease. Over the past few weeks, Cosmo has had increasing difficulty using his left hind leg. His vet noticed swelling of the limb, and X-rays revealed a mass. A biopsy was performed. Cosmo had already seen other veterinary specialists for this current cancer diagnosis, but his owners would not settle for the bleak news. I know his "mom," Laura Engel, who is also a veterinarian. We'd gone to different veterinary schools, then trained together while she was an intern and I was doing my oncology residency. That was many, many years ago, and I haven't seen her since. When she comes in with her husband, Eric, I give each of them a big hug. Then I reach down and pet Cosmo, who wags his furry golden retriever tail in greeting as he lies on the floor.

The husband and wife team give me a detailed history of their dog's condition, as they've already completed a workup, or battery of tests. Cosmo can no longer walk because he has histiosarcoma, a very aggressive type of cancer, which is eating through the bone of his stifle, or knee region. Due to his size and weight, the family use a red Flyer wagon to transport him around. It's cute to see, as long as you don't know the sad reason. It's also no way for Cosmo to live, and the Engels know that. Additionally, one of Cosmo's lymph nodes in his abdomen is a bit larger than it should be, so it's entirely possible that his cancer has already spread there. Then again, the lymph node may not have cancer in it and may merely be reactive, trying to keep the cancer at bay, albeit ineffectually. The Engels had been given the bad news, but they were waiting for me to offer some hope.

Hope is a tenuous thing. I always want to try to give a family hope that there are better days ahead, and that their pet will have a longer, healthier life. But I have to temper hope with realism. It does no one any good to be unprepared for what might lie ahead. Honesty, balanced with compassion, is my preferred path.

We speak at length about Cosmo's diagnosis. The Engels have no two-legged children. Cosmo fills that cherished role. He's the love of their lives, and they have had fourteen years of wonderful memories with him. For years, the trio has spent their Septembers hiking and swimming up in Maine. At least, Cosmo swam. The water is too cold in Maine for most non-Mainers to get in, but golden retrievers don't seem to care, and Cosmo would never miss a chance to splash in the ocean. The Engels see past all of Cosmo's other ailments. It doesn't matter to them that he's dealt with or currently is dealing with so many other issues. Up until this histiosarcoma, he has had a good quality of life. Cosmo is old, considered a geriatric in the veterinary world, especially for a large-breed dog. But age is not a disease, and so we consider his options.

The Engels understand that this type of cancer often progresses very quickly, so we review possible treatments. One option—though dismaying to the Engels—is amputation of the affected limb. As terrible as that sounds to us humans, many dogs left with only three legs do remarkably well, carrying on pretty much as usual. They run, catch Frisbees, jump up on the sofa, just as they could with four limbs. But Cosmo has had knee surgery on his other leg, which means that his "good" leg is not that strong. Compounding this problem is Cosmo's arthritis. He's on a host of medications that have helped him manage quite well until now. But removing a limb would put more weight on the remaining three, which would make his arthritic signs worse, and severely reduce his quality of life. Some dogs, when arthritis is terribly painful despite medications and even acupuncture, are humanely euthanized. As the Hippocratic Oath instructs us: first do no harm. For Cosmo, our goal is to improve his quality of life, not take away one problem only to replace it with another. And even with amputation, the golden's cancer could easily recur within just a few months. Understandably, the Engels decline this option.

A second possibility is radiation therapy, and I review the risks. Fortunately, cats and dogs do not get general "radiation sickness," meaning that there is no nausea, vomiting, or diarrhea. Side effects, when they do occur, tend to be limited to the area involved in treatment. For Cosmo, this means he might get a sunburn-like effect on his left leg. Topical medication can help, but the condition might take a few weeks to resolve. And it's possible that not all of Cosmo's fur will grow back. The fur that does regrow will come back white. But Cosmo wouldn't care about that.

As a human needing radiation, I have a much greater chance of getting an RT-induced burn. I see women in the changing room with bright red skin that looks incredibly sore. As I watch them gingerly remove their clothing, trying not to touch the painful area, my heart goes out to them. My doctor highly recommends that I put Eucerin cream on my RT site as a way to curtail these signs before they get too bad. After going to the drugstore and riffling through what seems like fifteen varieties of the emollient (who knew Eucerin had so many variations?), I buy the original, which is as thick as kindergarten paste. I call it my war paint. If I'm a soldier going into battle, I need my protective gear. I lather my abdomen up twice a day, every day, during these five weeks of radiation. I've been extremely fortunate and not sustained any cutaneous side effects. One bullet dodged.

For Cosmo, radiation means not needing any sort of surgery. He can keep all four legs, but some serious concerns remain. Even if treatment succeeds in reducing his cancer burden, it's possible that treatment will not restore his ability to walk. It is a dilemma deciding whether to put a pet through therapy and spend a great deal of money, not knowing how much he or she will improve. In Cosmo's case, the affected bone is already extremely weak, and the leg could simply break in two. This fracture could occur for no reason other than that the cancer has eaten through the bone. And treatment that can kill cancer cells in a very short period of time can also keep new healthy bone from having enough time to regenerate or grow. So, radiation could leave his leg more fragile than it is currently.

In exploring Cosmo's prognosis, the Engels and I know what will happen without any therapy, and we also know the risks associated with treatment. There's a chance that RT will not be of much benefit, and yet there's the chance that it could help for months. I've had some patients with this same disease do well for a year, and I've had some go the other way, fast.

When I asked my own doctors about my possible prognosis, no one gave me a number. No percentages, not one statistic. All three physicians were in unison, a well-orchestrated chorus, even though they didn't work out of the same wing of the cancer center. They told me numbers don't mean anything, that it only matters how I do. On a daily basis, I give out numbers: what percent have a chance of remission and for how long—in weeks, days, or months. Sometimes, I can say years. No matter the number, I tell the owners so that they understand what we're up against. Unrealistic hope is no gift. The families need to know what lies ahead, to know how much or how little time they have to spend with their pet. I can rattle off numbers like a savant. How else could we, as veterinarians, expect a pet parent to make choices, except by knowing the odds, the costs, and the risks that all go into a well-educated decision? But for me, the human patient, I get nothing. Goose egg. I'm told that numbers don't matter if you're part of the percent that's cured or that small percent that does poorly. Maybe they're right—better to go in with the best possible attitude. Pets always go in with the best possible attitude.

The Engels elect to proceed with radiation.

On the following Monday, Cosmo arrives at the vet center in his red wagon to begin his treatment plan. He will have a total of four appointments—the first for a CT scan. Computerized tomography will help us fully map his cancer, guiding us to sites we need the radiation to attack. Leaving out or missing any part of the cancer in the treatment area would be tragic—better safe than sorry—so we will include the enlarged lymph node. A vet tech anesthetizes Cosmo and places him in the CT machine. It takes less than an hour to obtain the necessary images. To ensure a consistent, reproducible, and precise setup, we create a mold of his hind quarters for him to lie in each time. On Wednesday, Cosmo will return to receive the first of three radiation doses, given on consecutive days.

When I go in for my radiation treatments, I always try to dress nicely, figuring that I should try to look good, even when I feel like hell. I'm not going to let the *C* word get the best of me. This is part of my battle plan. My husband, on the other hand, the man I love, dresses for extreme comfort when he comes with me, wearing the same dark blue sweatpants he wore to paint our first home in. Truth be told, and embarrassing as it is, I purchased those sweatpants sixteen years ago and wore them when I was pregnant. And now my dear spouse sports these speckled pants to interact with the outside world.

We sit in the waiting room each time, until the radiation therapy receptionist calls my name to head to machine 433. One day early on, I was wearing a pretty red dress, and Mike was wearing the infamous sweatpants with a long-sleeved T-shirt frayed at the neckline. The RT tech came up to us in the waiting room and leaned over to Mike.

"Excuse me, sir," the RT technician whispered, "I can help take you in for your treatment now." She gently offered her hand, thinking he was the cancer patient *and* needed assistance! I couldn't help but have an "I told you so" ear-to-ear smile. I would have thought the experience would have led him to retire the sweats, but alas, I was sadly mistaken.

Cosmo is still not able to walk on his own, so for his first treatment, the golden retriever comes in on a gurney. The Engels seem a bit nervous, especially after such a difficult decision, one that only makes sense if it gives their canine companion an improved quality of life. But will it? The technicians transfer the dog from his set of wheels to the radiation couch. The radiation table that a patient lies on is ironically called a couch. But this couch is far from comfortable.

Cosmo is with us for about forty-five minutes that Wednesday, then again on Thursday and Friday, completing his radiation protocol in a single week. He's a good patient who requires very little anesthesia to make him hold still. To ensure that we're targeting and treating not only the correct area, but *all* of the correct area, the pet is not supposed to move at all while the machine is on. A person going through RT can be expected to comply with this simple instruction, but a pet won't be able to stay perfectly still no matter how obedient.

When I undergo radiation treatments, I count in my head to pass the time. I thought I'd try to meditate, but that was way too ambitious The loud hum of the machine is too difficult to block out, and it causes me profound anxiety as I lie there with nothing more than a sheet over my naked body. As the unit rotates back and forth around me on the couch, I say in my head, "One thousand one, one thousand two, one thousand three . . ." I know that when I reach one thousand sixty-five, I'm done. Bam, the machine turns off. I'm sprung for another day.

Cosmo has no immediate side effects from his treatment. On Friday, his last RT session, the Engels wheel him back to their car in his red Flyer wagon, the radiation team giving a wave as the family pulls out onto the street. Oh, please let this work, I say, for Cosmo and for the Engels. But I know it will take time to see what the response, if any, will be.

By mid-September I have completed two weeks of my own

radiation therapy. It's no fun to have to commute into New York City every day—this would be true even if it were for a paycheck—yet having the companionship of one of my girlfriends who drive me in for each session has been lifesaving. Unfortunately, I develop some lower GI side effects. I've never before taken Lomotil, a tiny antidiarrheal pill, but this drug is fast becoming my bestie. I've joked that I've always wanted to be a size six, but not this way, and the doctors tell me how important it is to not lose weight. Most of my cat and dog patients end up gaining weight, because animals don't experience these same side effects, and no doubt people give their ailing pets extra treats. But with me, every doctor, nurse, radiation therapist, physician's assistant, informational handout, etcetera has told me how I need to maintain my weight during this process. Well, as an over-achieving rule follower . . . I've gained eight, yes, *eight*, pounds! I call them my "spares."

I receive a call from the Engels ten days or so after Cosmo's last RT. He's walking! It started with his trying to get up on his own and has progressed to slow steps. He needs the help of his people, and the Engels use a sling around his midsection to assist. This is very encouraging news so soon after treatment.

Two weeks out from RT, I see Cosmo back for his recheck visit. He has no pain, though at his treatment site he has no fur, but his skin is a nice, light pink-white. His knee has good range of motion, and the leg is much stronger, though it has sustained some muscle atrophy from not being used before he began treatment. However, the best news is that now Cosmo not only rises on his own, but readily walks around the house and yard without any assistance! The Engels were considering canceling their annual autumn trek to Maine, but in light of Cosmo's improvements, they decide to go, and bring Cosmo.

The Engels send me photos of Cosmo Down East, eagerly hiking on the beautiful, tree-lined carriage roads in Acadia National Park, decked out in their full autumn colors. Like a young dog, Cosmo walks ahead of his family, smelling and investigating, his golden blond against the backdrop of reds, oranges, yellows, and greens. I smile when looking at the pictures. The Engels were stunned and delighted when Cosmo bounded for the lake, then dove right in, swimming! They never lost hope, and they were rewarded by being able to add to their wonderful fourteen years of memories in their favorite vacation spot with their favorite companion.

Every couple of months, the Engels return with Cosmo so I can keep an eye on him. Early detection, whether for a person, cat, or dog, is of the utmost importance. Each visit, I perform a physical exam, run some screening blood work, and order up an abdominal ultrasound. Occasionally, we also might do chest X-rays. It takes about forty-five minutes to do all the things necessary to evaluate Cosmo, and waiting can be hard. Laura is well versed in all this, but I can sense her worry as I come back into the exam room. I give her a smile. All is good with Cosmo, and she breathes a sigh of relief.

I can relate. I will complete my radiation treatments this coming Monday. The cancer center has a large brass bell with a long, thick braided rope attached to the wall for their patients to ring at the conclusion of their RT protocol. I have seen (and heard) others do it when they're finished. Everyone claps and is genuinely happy for that individual. I've said that I do not want to ring the bell, because I won't be fully "done" until I complete more chemotherapy. But Mike, ever encouraging, wants to be there and see me ring that damn bell, signifying an end to this part of the journey. So, I'll do my bit. I'll ring it loud and proud!

The Engels take two trips to Maine, a year apart, with their beloved Cosmo. Periodically, they send me photos of happy moments. Cosmo with his birthday cake; Cosmo at Halloween; Cosmo holding his Christmas toy in his mouth. Cosmo has beaten the odds, staying in a remission for a full two years. It is these kinds of cases that help me do what I do.

"Call on line three, Cosmo Engel, line three," the reception-ist's voice echoes over the loudspeaker. I reach for the phone, looking forward to learning about Cosmo's latest escapade. But I can hear the bad news in Dr. Engel's voice the moment we say hello. She tells me that their boy had started limping a couple of weeks ago. At first, they thought he might have overdone it on a local hike, but rest and arthritis medications were of no avail. She took Cosmo into her clinic and X-rayed his leg.

"It's fractured," she blurts out. The gravity of her words hit me like a punch. My mind races and yet I am unable to form a coherent thought. We sit in silence, each of us on the opposite end of a cold, plastic phone receiver.

"Are you sure?" I ask, not wanting to believe my ears.

"Yeah, I had the surgeon and the radiologist review the rads. I don't know what I'm going to do." But we both know what she's going to have to do.

Sadly, at the age of sixteen, the golden retriever is experi-encing something that he won't be able to shake. The fracture Cosmo developed in his leg where the cancer had originated could be caused from recurrence of his histiosarcoma, weak-ening and eating through the bone. Or it could be due to a terrible, thankfully very rare side effect from his radiation treatment. The only way to know would be by anesthetizing him and performing a biopsy of his bone. However, the only truly helpful treatment for him at this time would be amputation of the affected limb, no matter the cause. It makes little sense to put Cosmo through a bone biopsy when it won't help him in the long run. Or even the short run.

Dr. Engel's voice descends into sadness.

"We always said our goal was him having the best quality of life," she begins. "We're so thankful for the two-plus years you gave us with our boy. He's had a great life. I don't know how I could ever repay you."

"The pleasure is all mine. I loved getting the photos you sent, seeing Cosmo's latest adventure. I wish it could have been longer, but he really did well for two years."

Given all of Cosmo's past medical problems, the arthritis, and his age, Dr. Engel tells me they will elect euthanasia. We hang up the phone but plan to stay in touch. As hard as it is to let go and say goodbye, the Engels don't want Cosmo to be in pain. They will have the procedure done in their home, where Cosmo is most comfortable and at ease. Upon hearing the news, Cassidy's eyes fill with tears. I remind her that Cosmo had such a good life, and two more years with excellent quality. I ask my tech if she'd like a hug, and she responds with wide, open arms. It is a very sad day for the family and for us at the clinic. We all love that boy and know he will be missed terribly.

4

DICKENS, DRUMMER, AND NEWTON

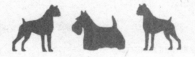

I decided to become a veterinarian in third grade, and I never wavered. Not once. Veterinary medicine has been and is a way of life for me; more than a job, more like a calling, or a duty. But I was never the kid who splinted the robin's broken little wing. In my defense, my mom wouldn't let me touch wild birds, saying they carried disease. I did stand diligently and watch my best elementary school friend as she tried to save a baby bird that had fallen out of its nest. I gave my opinions and advice, but as an avid rule follower, I did not touch that little chick.

In second grade, my parents got divorced. Our nuclear family of four turned into a single parent, my mom, alone with two young kids. It was not an easy time for her or us. An eternal dog lover, Mom was determined to get a dog to bring happiness to our new house.

Mom turned to her AKC breed book. She called friends and spoke with breeders, wanting to find a good fit. Months went by.

It was a long winter, and I made it longer by pining and begging for a dog. My mom had *promised*, after all, yet we had nothing. Then one spring day while walking home from second grade, I waved at our neighbor, who was working in her garden.

"Hi, Mrs. Green," I said.

"Oh, sweetie," she said. "You better hurry home quick! Your mom has a surprise for you!"

A dog! It must be a dog! I ran half a block as fast as my legs would take me. Bounding through the door, I dropped my backpack while shouting for my mom.

"I'm in here!" I heard her voice, but it was coming from the other side of the house. I ran down the hall to find my mom in my bedroom.

"You're painting my room?" I shouted in disbelief. "*That's* the surprise?!"

"Well, yes, I know you've wanted a pink bedroom, and I decided to begin."

"That's *not* a surprise," I replied, disappointment and belligerence oozing out of every pore. "Mrs. Green said it was a *surprise*."

"Ooh, you thought there was a different surprise? You mean a *puppy*?"

"Yeah."

"You should have gone to the family room first . . ."

"What?" My ears perked up. With that, I ran to the family room to find a little black Scottie puppy, safely tucked away in his dog crate. I opened the crate door as he wiggled out to me. His beard was tousled, like an old man with unkempt whiskers. I picked him up, instantly smelling his puppy breath. Holding him tightly, I felt so happy. Dickens, as we so aptly named him, was a good fit for our family. He was a scrappy dog whose place was right in the middle of a pack of kids, chasing a soccer ball in the backyard. We took him sledding on the hills at the local golf course during our cold Michigan winters. Little ice balls would dangle from the fur on his legs. Dickens's favorite pastime, though, was digging holes in the garden, which infuriated my mom. I proudly boasted that I taught our Scottie one command: how to sit up and beg. Though a one-trick pony, he knew how to coerce us into giving him a treat or a piece of leftover sandwich crust.

At the age of five, however, Dickens lost his spirited personality, became listless, and stopped eating much. Mom took him in to see the vet, who said that our dog had big lymph nodes. He called the condition lymphoma. This being the 1970s, prednisone was the only treatment that was offered. Back at home, Dickens continued to lie around, only I now lay with him, side by side on the carpet in the dining room, away from the flow of the household. I kept him company for days on end. After only a few weeks my mom took him to the vet's, but this time he didn't come back. I suppose that was my first experience with the dreaded *C* word.

I mourned Dickens for weeks. But once my grief subsided I really wanted another dog, and I decided to take matters into my own hands. Down from the shelf I pulled my mom's *The Complete Dog Book* from the AKC. I studied that book, reading up on the various breeds. I circled the ones I liked, crossed out the ones I didn't like. At last, I found my perfect breed: the boxer.

The Boxer: alert, dignified and self-assured, constrained animation, fundamentally playful yet patient and stoic, fearless courage, intelligent, loyal affection, makes him a highly desirable companion.
—AKC'S *THE COMPLETE DOG BOOK*

Spirited athlete, alert family guardian, arresting beauty (which) never fails to excite compliments as he trots jauntily by your side. Greatest wish is to be with the children, watching protectively, a "dog for all seasons." His strongest characteristic is his desire for human affection.
—THE AMERICAN BOXER CLUB

I wasn't quite sure what "jauntily" meant, but I knew I wanted that by my side. I begged my mom for a boxer. She was not on board. For weeks on end, I pleaded my case. Finally, we came to a compromise: I could get a boxer puppy if I saved up enough money to buy one myself. That was all I needed to hear. It took me months, but after numerous odd jobs and babysitting gigs I saved up enough money for a boxer puppy *and* a year's supply of food. My mom's jaw dropped when I told her of my "good" news—and true to her word, she drove me to pick out a boxer from a local litter of pups she found in the newspaper. We brought home an eight-week-old fawn male puppy, and my world was again made right. I named him Drummer. We bonded instantly.

Drummer was a bright spot and a lifeline. He brought security to me when my life felt insecure. With my mom working long hours, he was a steadfast friend who brought companionship, fun, and a sense of escape. Most importantly, Drummer was a creature who let me love him, and loved me right back, fully and completely. I've adored boxers ever since. It was my relationship with him that solidified that I had to be a veterinarian.

Boxers have been a prominent part of many life moments for me. They have even helped bring me love! Mike, my husband, is also a veterinarian, though he specializes in ophthalmology—diseases of the eye. We met twenty-five years ago, in New York City, when I was a resident and he was an intern. I remember the first time I saw him. I was leaving the hospital on a warm summer's evening, walking my boxer, Blitzen, when this guy caught my eye. He was of medium height, had medium brown hair, had a slender build, and was wearing khakis—just my type. Somehow seeing him made my heart beat a little faster. I thought, what a perfect opportunity, I'll walk Blitzen closer to him. Just as my dog stopped to sniff a small patch of green grass, I found myself staring at my newfound crush. Try as he might, this cute guy couldn't figure out how to cross the street! The oncoming traffic light would turn red. The lighted crosswalk sign flashed WALK! WALK! The streets were filled with yellow taxis and bustling cars, honking their horns. This twentysomething guy, sporting a large backpack, would step off the curb, his two suitcases rolling behind him, then *bam!* A car invariably would turn left into the crosswalk, causing my crush to scuttle back to the curb from which he came. This went on for several lights—he just could not get across. Just as I was about to head toward him to lend him a hand (or some New York moxie), I saw him readjust his backpack, then take a big deep breath as the crossing light signaled WALK! This time, determined to get across, he plowed on through and made it to the other side. I shook my head and smiled, realizing that I'd lost my chance to meet him. Oh well, Blitzen was a gift from a prior boyfriend; how could I expect my dog to lead me toward a new boyfriend? Besides, I needed

Blitzen to keep this midwestern girl grounded with the rigors of my residency program in the Big Apple.

The very next day, I was headed to the veterinary hospital's pharmacy after seeing my morning patients, and who should be right in front of me but the guy who'd been struggling to cross the street! He was in khakis again, this time with a clean, starched white lab coat. He was one of the new batch of interns who descended on the clinic that time of year. Despite having witnessed his crossing fiasco the previous day, I was nervous to talk to him. But the intern had an inviting smile and appeared kind. I welcomed him to the program and offered to be of assistance should he need it. I did not reveal that I'd witnessed his needing help navigating a New York City crosswalk! Though I couldn't put my finger on it, he felt very familiar. Turns out, Mike was from Kansas—I'd found another midwesterner in the middle of Manhattan.

Newton, our six-year-old brindle boxer, hangs with me as my constant nursemaid. I spend much of my time in our family room, where I've become a connoisseur of murder mysteries, under the tutelage of the good Ben Matlock and Lieutenant Columbo. Newton is a wonderful companion; his warm brown eyes look at me lovingly every day. When we got him as a pup, the breeder told us he was "special," which I thought odd because—aren't all puppies and kittens special? As he grew from eleven pounds into his adult body, slowly we understood what the breeder suspected. Newton never barks. Ring the doorbell, look like an intruder, still no bark. Boxers are by nature a working breed. In World War I, they were used as guard dogs, and they're supposed to bark, but Newton can't. He also doesn't always know when to stop drinking his water. He laps and laps and laps at the liquid in his bowl as the minutes go by. He still continues to drink until we say, "Hey, Newtie, stop." Turns out, he is mentally challenged. Seriously. I had him tested with an MRI, a magnetic resonance imaging scan, that showed that his brain isn't shaped the way a dog's brain should be. And it certainly doesn't sit in his skull correctly. What's more, he has a three-centimeter area that's missing from the middle of his brain. No tissue. Nada. Think donut. But I realize his "specialness" just makes us love him even more. He's sweet, goofy at times. We're totally devoted to him, and Newton is totally devoted to us. He doesn't care if I don't get dressed in the morning. He doesn't notice if my thinning, straggly chemo hair is plastered to my head. He doesn't judge me for lying on the sofa for days in a row. And we don't judge him for not barking at the door. Newton provides unconditional love for me and for my family, and we give him unconditional love right back.

Newton has once again assumed his position as steadfast

nurse, lying against the side of our dark blue sofa. I reach down to pet him, then hold my breath. Oh, please don't let it be. I spring to a seated position and feel again. The lymph nodes under Newton's neck are enlarged. Not huge, but definitely bigger than they should be. No, no, no, our dog cannot have cancer while I am going through my own battle. I'm terrified that this will be too much of a strain on our family, especially on our son. Peter is an only child, so Newton is like his younger brother. As much as Newton loves me, he is fully my son's dog.

I think about keeping this discovery to myself. Maybe I'm wrong. Maybe I'm overreacting. Maybe I'm limited by my veterinary oncology lens and think that cancer is the only possible explanation. Newton will need tests for us to be sure what's truly going on. What if this pushes my family over the edge?

I decide that I should tell my husband and son after all. Gentle but honest. I've found that it is better to prepare someone for what might lie ahead rather than hit them with the full wallop of bad news all at once. We are a family unit, and we should make these decisions together.

I pull myself off the sofa, and Newton gets up to go downstairs. For days I've been living in pajamas, but now I throw on a loose-fitting dress and slip into my Birkenstocks. I look at my hair in the mirror. It's definitely thinned, but it still covers all of my head. I'm told that no one notices but me, but I think people are just being nice. Oh well, staying alive is better than keeping a full head of hair. I go downstairs to find Peter and Mike in the kitchen. My teen is on his laptop at the breakfast table, and Newton has taken up a position under his chair.

"Hey, guys, I need to talk to you," I start off. Mike looks up from is coffee; he can hear from my tone that something is wrong. My son stops typing. I need to tread carefully now.

"I felt something on Newton that I think we should check out."

The color drains out of Mike's face. Peter slides off the chair and onto the ground, putting his arm lovingly around our dog's neck.

"I felt some big lymph nodes," I go on. "It might be nothing, but I'm worried it could be something worse . . . like cancer."

My husband knows what could lie ahead. We have had several boxers over the course of our relationship. We love the breed, even though they're afflicted with a fair amount of the C word. "Canines with the highest incidence of cancer" is not a list you want to sit atop, but I suppose I am one of those people who continue to do the same thing over and over, hoping for a different outcome. Sadly, some cancers are genetic in this breed, an anomaly that goes back for a good seven decades. If that's what this turns out to be, Newton would be our fourth boxer beset with the C word.

"Mom, how will we know?" Peter asks me. My sweet teenage boy. I love him so much. If I could shield him from having to know, I would. We all have to deal with issues growing up, but I would never want this for my child.

"I can do some tests to find out, honey."

"Well, we'll just have to treat him," Peter says. He pats the dog's head and adds, "It'll be okay, Newtie."

I'm holding back my tears. Deep breath. The three of us hug Newton, and then Peter and I start to cry. Mike even gets a bit misty. Before doing the tests, it's as if we all seem to "know."

Mike drives Newton and me to the clinic, though he stays in the car once we arrive. My husband prefers to keep a distance, letting me get to work. He says he doesn't know what to do to help, but I think it's all just too much for him. His wife and his dog. At the same time. Mike dampens his melancholy by reading and answering reams of emails on his phone. It serves as a good distraction.

I get out of the car and enter the gray brick building. My staff greets my dog and me with an inquisitive "Why are you here?" look.

I tell them what I've found as Newton wiggles his boxer rear end at record speed.

Sadness washes over the team, but they step up in their incredible way, which I've come to rely on every day of my professional life. Not only are they the backbone of my oncology service, but many a day, they're my own personal support system as well. Working together for years, we comfort each other when we have a sad case. We laugh together when we see a dog acting silly. We help each other as we share family issues. I care for them deeply. And through thick or thin, happy or sad cases, they always know I have their back.

My team is well versed in the drill, and they prepare for the tests. Though the table is set up to be about waist high at the moment, Newton leaps onto it with ease. He always perches on that green padded top like he's king of the castle when he gets to come to work with me. Today is no different. The height of the jump pulls us out of our somber mood, amazed at his agility and eagerness. The sadness lifts, at least for a moment.

The techs take two tubes' worth of blood to check Newton's white blood cell count, red blood cells, platelets, and organ function. In-house lab machines spit out the results in fifteen minutes. His blood work is fine, no issues there.

As my trusted coworkers take Newton down the hall to X-ray his lungs, I watch my beloved trot away. In another fifteen minutes, I'll have his results.

Thankfully, when I review the images, there're no signs of metastasis—no spreading—to the lungs. A deep breath. Two tests down, one to go.

Both Jackie and Cassidy gently hold my dog in a seated position while I take samples of his enlarged lymph nodes. This aspiration cytology is an easy test, like a reverse injection. I insert a needle into the lesion in question, then pull back on the plunger of the syringe, sucking out cells. No sutures needed, no bandages. The cells are put on glass slides, which are then packaged and sent to an outside laboratory for a pathologist to prepare with stain, then review under a microscope. It'll take two days to get the results. We will wait and try not to think about it.

The two days go by. I'm again back in residence in our family room—house arrest from chemotherapy. I have a *Matlock* playing on the television when I hear the ding of an incoming text. I reach for my phone and see that it's from one of my technicians, sending me the results. My dog has cancer. Lymphoma. I sit and stare for the next several minutes.

Confirmation of Newton's cancer hits me like a lead balloon. Recently, it's been too much for me to work while weathering the storm of my latest round of treatments. At times, the side effects are so bad that I can't get off the sofa for days. How in the hell will I be able to treat my dog?

I try to convince myself that I can somehow muster up the energy to drive Newton in for his treatments, once a week. Problem is, owing to my side effects, I haven't driven in weeks.

My cell phone dings again. As if they've picked up on the ramblings in my head, my friends (aka coworkers) offer to drive Newton to and from the clinic. Tears well in my eyes. How can I accept this kindness? But how can I not accept it? I am grateful to work with such wonderful people. I share the report and the offer of personal Uber service with my husband. I text the group back. We settle on a schedule of Mike's driving one way and a coworker the other, each time. I have no idea how I can repay the team's kindness, but I know one day I'll try.

The next morning, 6:00 a.m. sharp, a silver Honda pulls up in our driveway. Newton recognizes the veterinary nurse, and he goes into a full rear end wiggle as he heads across the lawn and hops into her car. Always happy to go for a ride, the boxer is completely unsuspecting. The technician looks back at me, trying to hide her sorrowful eyes with a warm smile. But I feel her sadness just the same.

Once at the veterinary hospital, Newton walks onto the scale and they check his weight. I receive a text telling me this information so that I can calculate his correct drug dosage. I text back with instructions for his first treatment. I am not there to be with or help my boy, but my team does what they do best. I trust them completely.

On his way back from work at the end of the day, Mike brings Newtie home. You wouldn't know that anything has changed. The boxer trots to his food bowl to see if dinner has miraculously appeared, then sniffs the empty container. I pick up the white ceramic bowl and fill it with his favorite kibble, which he gobbles down before asking to go outside.

Newton appears unfazed by his first day of chemotherapy, yet my own recent treatments have been much more taxing. I sit in the hospital bed for eight and a half hours with an IV stuck in the top of my hand. Once I get home, I am usually down and out for about four and a half days, generally alone—Mike at work, Peter at school—except for Newton, who is my steady partner.

I wasn't planning on side effects I couldn't handle, but then I was hit with really severe bone and joint pains. Hurting, I swallowed my pride and asked a girlfriend to stop by to rub my legs. Never in a million years did I think I'd ever be asking a friend to provide that kind of nursing care, but that's how bad the pain is. Dignity goes out the window when you really need help.

The cancer center nurse tells me this side effect will go away, but it can take a long time, like a year. *A year!*, I think. If it really lasts that long, I'll do my best not to complain, but the pain really limits me. I worry that I won't make it through three more of these treatments, and I can understand why some people give up. The saving grace, though, is the realization that, with each treatment, I'm that much closer to being done. This week I need to will up my white blood cells, platelets, and red cells. "Mind over matter" as a therapeutic intervention. It's a full-time job, and it takes a lot of energy.

Six days after Newton's first treatment, I pad down to the kitchen, still in my loungewear. Mike and Peter are scarfing down breakfast before heading out for their day. They put down their forks and watch as I examine Newton—feeling all his lymph nodes, palpating his belly, listening to his heart and his lungs. You could hear a pin drop, aside from the hum of the morning television news show on in the background. I stand up and smile. Newton's left the rest of us C word patients in his dust! He's gone into a complete remission with his very first dose of chemotherapy and, so far, without a single side effect—a very positive step. Newton's motto seems to be: "What cancer? What chemo?" I admire his attitude. We could use some good news, and my family and I shout in joy. Newton jumps around even though he does not realize why we're celebrating.

"C'mon, boy, let's go for a walk," Mike says as he heads to get Newtie's leash. The dog, eager as always, spins around in little circles.

"Don't you have to get to work?" I ask, glancing at the clock on the oven.

"I'm okay, I have a few minutes," Mike replies with a grin. Taking a walk through the neighborhood with Newton is one of my husband's favorite things. I smile to see them both happy, heading out for their time together.

My dog begins to wait by the door for his rides, as if he has the car pool written down in his daily planner. Each week my oncology team sends me a picture of his blood work results and his current weight, and I text back his dose. Somehow, while I'm struggling to keep my food in, my dog is packing on the pounds.

The night before each of Newton's scheduled treatments, I perform the same physical examination on him. At the beginning, I'd hold my breath until I felt all of his lymph nodes, confirming that he was, in fact, still in a remission. Weeks go by, and he continues to do well. After two months, Newtie continues to take his new schedule in stride, and I come to expect that each time I examine him, his lymph nodes will be normal. No more bated breath. Then, three months to the day since his diagnosis, I bend down to do my usual evaluation, and I feel it. Mildly enlarged lymph nodes. Newton's cancer is back. It's not a good sign that it's returned so quickly. In general, the protocol he's on should have kept his disease in check for a full year. I guess his cancer had other plans.

I tell my family my findings but try to relay it in a way that makes it sound routine. Fortunately, I still have a few more tricks up my sleeve. Peter gives me the side eye, not really sure if he should believe me. I chalk it up to being a teen. Mike, on the other hand, is adept enough to realize what this means. I try to disguise my worry with a weak smile. I know that the cancer's rapid return is a sign that it's aggressive and resistant. I stifle those thoughts with Girl Scout cookies. Thin Mints. Frozen. The best therapist in town.

The next morning, I call the oncology technicians to brief them on my findings. I choose a different protocol. Newton will have to receive his intravenous medication over five hours. But he's very accustomed to being at the vet clinic all day, waiting for Mike to retrieve him. Newton's chariot arrives at seven, and he goes off in the car like it's any other day, happy to be a dog.

Once he arrives, a tech places an intravenous catheter in his vein and hooks up the chemo bag, and the five-hour countdown begins. I think about him a lot while he's there and I'm home, beneath a blanket, under house arrest.

That evening, Newton comes back a bit tired from his day. He eats his kibble without his usual enthusiasm, makes a quick trip to the backyard to do his business, then tucks into his dog bed. I watch him intently, but I don't want to alarm my family. It seems that my chemotherapy is working for me, and I wait and hope that his will work for him.

As the week goes by, Newton sleeps more, though he's in good spirits. I'm not sure my family notices his apparent fatigue. They've grown accustomed to our dog being by my side while I'm convalescing. I refrain from feeling Newtie's lymph nodes until I can't hold back any longer—a whole five days.

His swellings are softer and a bit smaller. We're going in the right direction, albeit with baby steps.

Three weeks go by and Newtie is due for his second treatment. If this works, he'll receive a five-hour treatment once every three weeks, for a total of five sessions. And he's already had one of those five.

After our family dinner, I have him assume his position in the kitchen, standing still for his physical exam. Mike and Peter look at me in anticipation, searching my face for telltale signs. Mike could do a physical exam on our dog. After all, he is a trained, licensed vet. But he chooses to let me do it; he'd rather not know than know. I can't say that I blame him. And he is doing a remarkable job holding us all up. Sometimes I don't want to know, too, but my urge for the truth always wins out.

"Well, how do they feel?" Peter asks. "Is he okay?" I can hear the quiver in his voice.

"He's doing okay," I say. "The lymph nodes have decreased about fifty percent. They're definitely better, though they're not yet normal." I feel both sets of eyes on me. "And tomorrow he's due for his second treatment. And that should help his nodes go down even further. "

"C'mon, Newtie," I say. "Let's go upstairs and get some rest. We both need to be strong for tomorrow." And with that, the *C* word patients head up to bed.

At 6:00 a.m. the following morning, Newton and I are standing by the front door, each waiting for his or her ride. They say a dog is a wonderful companion for anything—I just never thought we'd be going through this particular journey together. Fortunately, I have girlfriends to be my companions through this as well. As the silver Honda Accord pulls up, the dog and I head out the door. Newton eagerly jumps into the back seat, heading to my office for blood work and chemotherapy. He's never had an issue with his blood, and ideally, today will be no different. If there's a problem, it will be hard for me to amend his plan remotely, while undergoing my own treatment.

I head back into the house, into the kitchen to futz until my friend Kate gets here. Aimlessly, I move some plants a few millimeters here, a few millimeters there. I spray the counter with some cleaner, then rub haphazardly to wipe up the liquid. I have experienced good, improved days, but now I face going through the cycle again, feeling sick from treatment. My stomach gurgles in nervous anticipation while thinking back to my very first chemo. Even though I'd administered the treatment to animals for more than twenty-five years—maybe *because* I'd administered the treatment for so long—I had a bit of a breakdown right before that very first session, as dread flooded my body.

I also felt that the cancer center didn't adequately brief me on what the day would be like; nor did they say enough about the possible side effects. Given all that I knew, I had a magnifying glass on all of those risks you see in the fine print of a commercial for a medication that seems worse than the condition it's meant to treat. And I wanted answers.

Mike accompanied me to that first treatment. This meant that my husband had to witness my reaction to the IV nurse as she so innocently entered the room to place my intravenous catheter. With my heart pounding, I began a long rant in a loud voice: "Which vein are you going to use? How long will the infusion take? When will the side effects start? How sick is sick? When should I call for help? Do you give me pre-medication before the actual medication? What if the chemotherapy leaks out of my vein? What if I need to go to the bathroom? Isn't anyone going to do a complete physical exam on me before I get this stuff? Will I be in pain . . ."

The nurse looked at me in bewilderment, glanced at Mike, then rushed out of the room. Mike gave me those spousal eyes that say "shut the bleep up," but I wasn't about to be stifled. I wasn't refusing treatment, I wasn't being rude—at least not intentionally—I simply needed information. But what I really needed was for someone, anyone, to quell my fears. Thankfully, the center was very skilled at handling my kind of panic.

The nurse returned with a very calm, reassuring physician's assistant in tow. The PA patiently answered my gunfire list as

I glared at Mike with a "see-I-told-you-so" look. I felt entirely justified for my outburst, and I'm sure I wasn't their only patient to lose it on their first day. I did, however, apologize to the nursing staff and to Mike.

From the kitchen, I hear my girlfriend's car round our circular drive. Kate has taken the day off from life, from work, from her family, to drive me to the cancer center. She will sit with me for as long as it takes to get my blood work done and to receive the eight and a half hours of treatment. She will be my "Newton" today.

I come out to the car and Kate gives me a big hug. She knows I'm nervous, but we don't speak of that. Instead, we get in and buckle up and begin talking about our kids, about the school they both attend, about the assignments they missed turning in. We talk about our husbands, the latest books we're reading, the TV shows we're watching. The subject doesn't matter, because mostly we talk to connect, to bond us together, to help keep my mind from dwelling on the day ahead or the what-ifs.

Kate does her darndest to keep things upbeat, but despite our steady banter, I can tell that even she is a bit nervous. Unsure what the day may hold, unsure how I will be, Kate does her best to conceal her feelings, but we have been friends for a long time. I can tell what's going on without the need for words. I guess that goes both ways, and she knows my brave face is masking a lot of anxiety.

It takes about fifty minutes to get to the hospital. Just before we pull up to the parking garage, my phone dings. It's a text of Newtie's blood work. I look at it, then close my eyes. Normal. Thank you. I quickly text my team back with gratitude and instructions to proceed with his treatment.

Being a fretter, I worry that today's treatment for me will worsen the aural side effects I've been experiencing. I have been having terrible tinnitus, or ringing, in my ears. I swore from the start that I'd simply use willpower to deflect any side effects, as if I had superpowers. The risk of nausea, vomiting, and diarrhea, or a low white blood cell count—these I was prepared for. However, I forgot that one of the drugs in my cocktail can cause ear issues.

I have an appointment with an ENT specialist to assess my ears before this scheduled chemotherapy. They will examine both ears and will perform a hearing test while we wait for my blood work results. Hope springs eternal, and my hope is that it's an ear infection.

Entering the cancer center, I see one of the senior nurses—Nurse Q, they call her—across the waiting room. She's been on my team before, and I nod while giving her a big smile. I feel more secure knowing that she's here.

Kate and I sit in silence, though trying to fill the void with small talk, but my mind is racing with I hope my blood work is okay, I hope my ears will be fine, I hope my chemo goes smoothly. If I were giving advice to someone else, I would point out that all this brooding is a waste of energy. I've confirmed the benefits of lack of worry, treating my cat and dog patients over many years. But even the most ingrained lessons can be hard to apply to one's own situation, and right now, this one's beyond my grasp.

I look around. The large waiting room is full. So many people coming here each day, waiting like I am for what they hope will cure them, or at least keep their cancer at bay. Most are sitting with a spouse or a friend. A few seem to have brought the whole family. Thankfully, very few are alone. But each of us has his or her own way of going through this. Today, my method is with anxiety.

When they call my name, my friend stays with our coats and purses in the waiting room. I look back at her, and she gives me an encouraging smile.

The process begins with a blood draw, and I pray the venipuncturist can get a clean, easy stick. Thankfully, she nails it on the first try. She then asks me to step onto the scale to record my weight. I swear this is the first time in my life I've wanted to keep on all clothes, including my shoes, while being weighed. In the past I would have played any angle to be as light as I could. One time, I asked the nurse to subtract three pounds because I was wearing boots. But in fighting the C word, a few extra pounds are a gift.

With normal blood work and no ear infection diagnosed, I am set for my next round of chemotherapy. Kate is by my side as I settle into the hospital room, ready to have a catheter placed for the treatment to begin.

When I arrive back home, the family is all there, Newton included. Mike can see how drained I am, but he acts upbeat in a show of support, greeting me at the door with a big hug. He is a sight for sore eyes, though I can tell he is wiped out as well. Peter is upstairs doing his homework, or so I hope. Newton is a bit off to the side, which tells me that his day has been tiring as well. Mike has dinner waiting for me: pasta. He is no fool; he knows my comfort food of choice. Handing me my plate, Mike plants a kiss on my forehead. As I sit at the kitchen island to eat, I hear the click of Newton's toenails as he goes upstairs. He sleeps in his dog bed until morning.

5

NEWTON, PART TWO

N eeewton!" I shout out the back door. My dog is in a stand-off with our neighbor's calico cat. I'd left him outside in our fenced-in yard for a few minutes, unattended, so he could sunbathe. Given that he's a dark brindle boxer, we say that he's "working on his stripes" when he sleeps in the sun. This dog loves the sun, but right now he's cornered an overconfident or perhaps over-curious cat. "Newton *come!*" I say in my sternest voice. The dog looks back at me, weighing his options. Which is the greater good—keeping this cat out of his backyard, or listening to his mom? "NEWTON!" I shout. The neighbors must think I've lost my marbles. The dog runs inside. He knows Momma means business.

Newton's second five-hour chemotherapy treatment a

couple of weeks ago has further reduced his lymph nodes, and he's been holding his own. Judging from the vigor he showed in facing down his nemesis the cat, I'd say he's feeling pretty good. I'd still prefer to see his lymph nodes all be normal, but at least they're going in the right direction, and for that I'm grateful. With my days shaping up to be more of a struggle than I anticipated, I'll take what good news I can get.

I sit down at my computer at the kitchen table. I have been using email to keep in touch with friends and family. I can't bear to have all the conversations be about me, so I write everyone in one big group to update them on where I am in the treatment process, and how I'm feeling. I end the email with:

I want to thank you all again for your unyielding support. I am astounded by your incredible love and caring. You help get me through this process and make it so much better than anything I could ever imagine. I am grateful that you are in my life. There are times that I don't know why you are all so kind, but I know enough to just say thank you. As always, thank you for being the best army a girl could ever ask for. xo, Renee.

"Hi, Mom," Peter shouts as he and a friend arrive home from school. I shut my computer. The boys make a pile of backpacks and unworn jackets on the floor next to the front door.

"We're gonna go shoot some hoops out back," he informs me. "C'mon, Newtie," he says as the trio heads out the back door. I check quickly—no more cat in sight. Newton jumps and dodges the large orange ball as the game starts up in our driveway. Both boys are laughing as Newton inserts himself into their one-on-one, and it warms my heart. Despite his chemotherapy, Newtie always seems to show up for his family, and I know it helps my son. I hope I've shown up enough for my family during my battle and not simply drained them and dragged them down. I've been there for the big things, though I'm not so sure about the little things.

Mike has shouldered the household chores while simultaneously being the main breadwinner. Before, when everyone was "healthy," he and I were more like two ships passing in the night, trying to balance independent work lives with the rigors of family life. Being in the same profession, we understand how the demands of veterinary medicine, a job we both love, can be all-consuming. I just wish we could have taken a pause—time to breathe, time for us—for our own sakes before having to deal with this life lesson. And now in order to keep things going, much has fallen on Mike, and he is holding up well, though at times I can see the strain in his weary eyes.

Peter navigates school, as well as his after-school activities, without any real guidance from me. I don't want to let him down, yet I console myself thinking that there's value in his learning to manage for himself. In times past, his "I got this," or "Don't worry about it," would cause me to do just that: worry, big-time. Now I'm proud to see our teenager stepping up just when we need him to.

This weekend, Mike will be away in Boston for work on a pharmaceutical consulting job, and I'm a bit concerned, mostly because I don't want to be a burden on Peter or on any of my girlfriends. I want my son to just get to be a kid, or really an adolescent, and not have to worry about me. I can try to manage things on my own, but my stamina isn't what it used to be, and sometimes I just feel rotten the whole damn day. But I'll take it slow, and rest when I need to rest. I'll also order a lot of pizza to be delivered—every teenager's dream.

I spend a lot of hours resting in the family room over the two days. Peter peeks his head in periodically, and I tell myself it's to make sure I'm okay. But what if it's to see if I'm awake enough to catch him at whatever he's up to? In actuality, his checking in makes me feel good. I feel loved, and I know that as self-centered as teenagers can be, Peter caring for things outside himself is a sign we must be doing something right.

On Sunday, I hear him start the washing machine. Now I'm worried. This is a boy who keeps his dirty clothes and his clean clothes in the same big heap on his bedroom floor. What's happening? I'm supposed to be the mom, the person who washes his clothes. Taking care of him actually gives me joy, yet I'm lying like a lump on the sofa. I will myself up, slowly padding into the laundry room. Though I'm so immensely proud of him, I hear myself say, "Here, let me do that."

Monday morning comes around faster than anticipated. Amazing how weekend time is always faster than weekday time. Tomorrow, Newton is due for his next chemotherapy. Today, I'll need to confirm his ride and check his lymph nodes. Newton's been doing well at home, though he's sleeping a little more than usual. Then again, so am I. Newton actively engages with Peter when he is home from school and wants to play. Otherwise, our boxer hangs by my side like my own private nurse.

"Hey, am I driving Newton this week?" Mike asks, coming into the kitchen for his essential cup of coffee first thing. My husband arrived home from his business trip late last night and I feel relief that he's home.

"Yes, I'm surprised you're asking. You usually forget until I remind you. No offense," I say, as I throw him a flirty smile.

"Weeell," he starts out.

"Well, what? You can still do it, right?" I can't ask any more people to drive our dog.

"No, no, I can drive him. It's just that, well, I think they're back," he explained. He glances at me with a "don't shoot the messenger" look. I feel a knot in the pit of my stomach. I hope Mike is wrong.

"Newtie, come here, honey," I tell our boy.

I feel his lymph nodes, this time starting from his back end and working my way up to his head, as if reversing my typical evaluation will give me a better result.

"Dammit," I say under my breath. Out of ten lymph nodes, seven are enlarged. And what adds insult to injury is that his liver is enlarged, whereas in the past, it's been normal. As the cancer progresses, it can easily spread to both the liver and the spleen.

I'm scared to death. The plan was that Newton and I would both get through this together. Is this a bad omen for me? I love Newtie so much, his warm brown eyes, his wrinkly face looking up at me. This isn't about me, I tell myself, but I need him. Why does he have to have such a persistent, resistant cancer? How can I cushion this for our son?

I don't know the answer, but I do know we shouldn't tell Peter before he heads off to school this morning. No reason to have him worry throughout his day. Mike and I both agree to that.

After Peter and Mike have headed off, I decide to text my work team to give them a heads-up for a new plan for Newtie, beginning tomorrow. It makes no sense to keep with the same protocol—it's obviously not doing the trick. I want him to begin a different cocktail of medications his cancer cells have not yet seen. This will give us a 50 percent chance of putting him back in a remission. If he were "average" (and we already know he isn't), it should keep him in a remission for up to a year. Fingers crossed. I instruct my team to do the usual blood work and to weigh him, then to text me for the dose calculations. Fortunately, my own chemotherapy isn't scheduled for another couple of days, so I can focus my attention on my dog. Still, I have to go to the cancer center to have some preliminary tests. I have three CT scans scheduled, one brain MRI (for the ringing in my ears), four blood tests, another hearing test . . . and a partridge in a pear tree. On a good day, I tell myself that the ringing is my body reminding me to be grateful for my life. On a not-good day, it's an invitation to a pity party. I just hope it won't affect my hearing. I head upstairs to put on some comfortable but presentable clothes for my busy day.

At 5:45 the next morning, the ringing in my ears is my incessant phone alarm. Ugh. I'm exhausted, both emotionally and physically. Yesterday's tests were a lot to do in one day, and the barrage really took it out of me. Perhaps I was overzealous, but I prefer one day of too many tests to having multiple days eaten up with coming and going. This is my time, and at least I get to have some control as to what I do with it.

On top of crushing fatigue, the stress of the what-ifs concerning my impending results is weighing on me. My body feels heavy and slow, but I need to get out of bed to get Newton ready for pickup. The dog lifts his head from his dog bed. Mike continues to snore even with the annoying alarm. I know he's exhausted as well. I pivot around and slowly put my two feet on the floor. This is going to be one of those not-so-good days.

Newton and I pad downstairs. He knows the drill. I let him

outside, and while he is attending to his morning business, I put his breakfast in his dog bowl and freshen his water. When I let him inside, he heads for the bowl, but slowly. No running, not today. Ideally, the chemotherapy will put a spring back in his step. Despite his slowness, Newton licks his bowl clean, and I wipe his moist jowls. (He's still my baby.)

"Good boy," I praise while rubbing behind his ear. He always loves this spot. I get Newton's leash and hook it to his collar, and he's ready and waiting by the front door. I head back to the kitchen to pour myself a glass of milk. Just then, a car pulls into the circular driveway and Newton begins to whine in anticipation. Recognizing his ride, he starts to pace back and forth. I run to settle him at the door—I don't want to wake the rest of the household. Good-natured as always, Newton eagerly goes to my colleague, then tries to hop onto the back seat. Today, he needs a little help up with his hind legs. I can see Newton's big pink boxer tongue hanging out of his mouth as the two drive away.

Within the hour, my team texts me Newton's blood work results and his current weight. He's slightly anemic but otherwise holding his own. I text back, sending them doses for the new plan, and I know they'll do their best.

Mike and Peter leave for work and school, and with a cup of black, decaffeinated tea in hand, I head to the family room sofa to lie down. Today is a rest day. Pulling a blanket up to my neck, I say a small prayer that this chemo protocol will work for our sweet dog. I find a *Columbo* on our DVR and fall into a deep sleep to yet another episode. What feels like a short time later, I awaken to hear the sound of the key going into the lock on the front door. It is 5:00 p.m.! How did I sleep away an entire day?

I throw off the blanket, then head to greet my three guys as they tromp into the house. Mike has made the rounds to pick up Newton after the dog's treatment and to get Peter from after-school band. And I have done nothing to help our household. I feel bad, but I do know that my body must have needed some major downtime. I suggest we order pizza, and both my two-legged boys are all smiles.

I'm hell-bent on staying on schedule, and fortunately, the next day I feel moderately stronger. My hearing test, thankfully, showed that all was good—no loss of function. My doctors say that the pain and tinnitus (ringing) will improve once chemotherapy is over, although it may take many months, and may never go away completely.

On a positive note, I still have my "mom ears," the auditory equivalent of having eyes in the back of your head. This should enable me to continue to pick up and foil my kid's nefarious plans and detect other information he may not want me to know. Even so, I will have the hearing test repeated two days prior to each chemotherapy treatment, just to make sure. And because my lab tests are all fine, my treatment will stay on schedule.

This time it is Harper who picks me up in her car for the ride into the treatment center. It's a bank/government holiday, so we make record time. I can tell she's nervous, talking nonstop, at full speed. I've lost track of the number of run-on sentences; I know this is her response to anxiety. I put my hand on her arm, and a tear rolls down her face. We enter the cancer center and I hear her sigh. I, on the other hand, am geared up. It is as if a switch has been turned on with the onset of Newton's treatment. I'm standing tall—an authoritative figure—as I check in at the reception desk. This is my war, and I will win this battle. I will fear no evil.

"Nurse Q, bring it on!" I say as she enters my room. She looks at me like I'm crazy. Good thing I had a brain MRI two days ago—I can prove I'm not completely deranged.

In my efforts to practice self-care, I bring a prerecorded meditation to play. The staff at the center probably think I'm a bit over the top, but of all the struggles in my life, this is probably as good a time as any to go for broke. Harper knows I march to the beat of my own drummer, or in this case, the beat of the meditation lady. Prior to the C word, I maybe did a five-minute meditation from a free app on my cell phone a couple of times a month. Maybe. But now, I have a therapist who records a fifteen-to-twenty-minute guided meditation for me to play each time as the chemotherapy begins to enter my veins. The first time I did it, Mike was with me. When the meditation stopped, I opened my eyes and noticed my husband asleep, head bobbing on his chest! Today, as Nurse Q starts my lengthy IV chemotherapy drip, I press the play button on my phone. I close my eyes and allow myself to tune out everything but the soothing voice:

Let's begin by placing your hand over your heart, or have your arms rest comfortably by your sides. We will start by taking three deep breaths in, holding each, then letting each one out slowly. And when we visit each organ, we want to bring gratitude to each and every one of them. Feel the compassion and support in a warm, golden, molten, healing, light energy flowing in you. We will begin at the bottom on your left foot. See if there is any sensation there . . .

The sweet sounds lead me softly. When the meditation is finished, I slowly open my eyes. Nurse Q has stayed with me the entire time! She smiles a big smile, pats my leg, then walks out of the room.

Each time I receive chemotherapy, the ringing in my ears changes pitch and tone. Right now, the music isn't all that bad. We don't know if cats and dogs experience this same side effect, but it wouldn't surprise me if they did with a couple of the drugs we use. While there's no way to test their ears for ringing, and our pets can't use words to tell us, I've never had a pet parent report a change with regard to an animal's ears. With ear pain, however, the animal would shy away when a person came near, or they might shake their head, and/or they might whine in discomfort. Thankfully, I haven't seen that in the patients I treat.

After Harper drops me back at home, I'm down for the count once again, feeling nauseated and listless for several days. Then, as per usual, I rally for a couple of days, but then the bone and joint pains begin again, and the lethargy returns. I'm told that I am weathering this well, though I have no basis for comparison, aside from my four-legged patients. Only two more rounds to go, but from my vantage point, two seems like an enormous number.

Days meld together as Newton and I spend time at home. It's day six since he received his new chemotherapy treatment, and he's due for another round tomorrow. At this point, I don't want to feel his lymph nodes, because I don't want to know if the news isn't good. It's all a bit too difficult today. In fact, I know I really just need to cry about it. Usually, the waterworks flow freely. Today I can feel the tears in my eyes, but I hold them back. I tell myself I should be exuding positive energy, but that's extremely hard to do when the crying starts. Additionally, I don't want to bring down Mike or Peter. Deep breaths. Trust that both Newton and I will be just fine. Today is a no-makeup day (they all are of late), so I really have no excuse not to cry. But my wall is up like a fortress in this battle. I know I'd feel better if I let it all out, but that's just not me right now.

By evening, I know I can't put off examining Newton any longer. Mike is at his desk, doing work with the Chiefs' football game on television in the background. My husband and I both know he's more engaged with the game than with whatever is staring back at him from his computer. He will be there for hours. Our teenager is upstairs, writing the term paper—please God—that's due in two days. From a boy's perspective, that's loads of time. From my viewpoint, it seems late already.

"Come here, Newtie," I say to our boxer. The dog walks over to me, giving a faint wag of his stub of a tail. He knows something's up as I reach for his lymph nodes, this time heading straight under his neck, then working my way down. Next comes palpating his abdomen, then listening to his heart and lungs with my stethoscope.

"Oh, thank goodness," I say with a sigh. I hug Newton around his neck. This *C* word is an emotional roller coaster, but it may be that we hang on for the "ups" all the more, knowing about the "downs" that inevitably follow. One tear escapes my lower lid, and my dog licks my face. I can't help but smile.

"Miiike. Peeeter," I shout. Nothing. I shout their names again, and this time they both come into the kitchen. "Newton's cancer is doing better," I say in a calm, measured voice.

"So the chemo's working, Mom?"

"So far, yes. But it is early yet." We've been fooled by this before; I don't want to encourage false hopes in either of my guys. "Hopefully, this protocol will hold him for a while." I smile, then hug my son tight. I smell his head, so I can get a good mom fix. Just as we're embracing, Newton shakes his head and his slobber goes flying.

"Eeew!" Peter lets out, along with peals of laughter. The dog still has a long, ropey bit of saliva hanging from his left jowl. It gets longer by the second. Boxers!

"What are we going to do with our Newtie?" Mike says fondly. Normally, Mike would complain about the drool, but tonight he's happy to clean up the mess. Tonight, we're all happy to have our dog with us, slobber and all.

"This calls for a walk! Wanna go on a walk, Newtie-Putie?" Mike asks eagerly. Newton breaks into his happy circle dance as Mike struggles to get the leash around the moving target that is our dog's neck.

The next morning, Newton is chauffeured to my office as

per usual for his next treatment. The blood work forwarded to me shows that his anemia has improved. Bam! Two steps in the right direction, lymph nodes and red blood cells.

That evening, Mike brings him home, and Newton runs to his food bowl, just in case that vessel has filled miraculously on its own, but he finds not a morsel. Newtie spins in a little circle by his bowl in eager anticipation. When his dinner comes, he gobbles it down. After his obligatory trip outside, we all head upstairs to tuck in early. All is right with our pup—all is right with our world. Tonight the household is peaceful and happy.

Four months into his protocol, one of Newton's lymph nodes decides to enlarge. His other lymph nodes palpate normally, though, so I'll keep a watchful eye but not change anything as of yet. Newton continues to receive his chemotherapy and seems to be feeling well.

But after another couple of weeks, I can't deny it any longer. His cancer is progressing, and I can feel his lymph nodes enlarging underneath his neck and in his shoulders. When Newtie turns his head a certain way, I can actually see the bulges. Why is it that the shoemaker's children wind up with no shoes? I have only one more protocol left to try on him, a chemotherapy pill that has potentially more side effects than his previous injectable drugs. In addition to stomach upset, this new protocol has a 6 percent chance of causing liver or kidney failure. Those odds are quite small, but my dog has never followed the law of averages. Still, we have to play the hand we're dealt.

6

BOGART

My technicians and I have seen and treated eighteen cases with two more to go. We're all exhausted, but we know we've made a difference in the lives of animals and the families who love them. To help us get through the day, we put on music. I am partial to eighties; my team wrestles to control the channel between hip-hop and country. The music puts a spring in each of our steps.

I am so grateful to be back at work. With the effects of chemotherapy getting easier, my strength and stamina are returning, albeit more slowly than I'd like. But I no longer complain about long, draining days at work. Despite today's office marathon, it is as if I am seeing all this with new eyes. I am blessed to feel good enough, be healthy enough, to work, but sometimes being both a patient and a clinician is hard. My emotions are still raw when I talk about a new animal's cancer to a pet parent during the initial consultation. It's all a bit too close to home, but I can't change that. All I can do is soldier on to fight that dreaded C word—whether for myself or for a trusting animal.

Sitting in my office, I muse about the little black and tan Yorkie who'd graduated from radiation therapy years ago, who came in to see me this morning. Stella peeked out of a Gucci purse, with a small pink blanket wrapped around her. Her owner was frantic, convinced that the dog's tumor had recurred. I unwrapped Stella from her soft leather carrier and warm blanket, then examined the area in question. Parting her fur, I could see that the lesion was about five millimeters in size, brownish in color, on the outer part of her thigh. I looked up with a big smile on my face: the dog had a tick. The lady's jaw fell open. It happens all the time, especially after a scary diagnosis. I can relate all too well.

I went to the dermatologist not long ago, convinced that I had cutaneous melanoma. I noticed a deeply black "mole" on the midsection of my abdomen. The dermatologist gave my bare belly a keen look through her magnifying glass, and as she glanced up at me, I could see she was stifling a little chuckle. That "mole" was a radiation therapy tattoo. The cancer center RT tech used this to help properly align the radiation machine to my body for each session. I understood how

Stella's mom felt, but I didn't chuckle. I was just so glad to be able to relay good news.

Sometimes a diagnosis comes as a total shock and surprise. Sometimes, like with Stella the Yorkie, we believe something is wrong . . . when everything is actually fine. Other times, our animal instincts tell us something isn't right, and we just *know*.

I pick up the chart to review for my next appointment. Combing through the records, there is no diagnosis of cancer that I can find. Hmm, maybe I should call the referring vet to see if there are some results that we may be missing.

As I enter the exam room, I am met with a woman in her mid-fifties. She is pacing a bit, while biting at the cuticle on her nail. Her dark, wavy hair comes down to the middle of her back. I am greeted by her overly eager golden retriever. Gus is a seven-year-old male dog who within seconds puts his two bear-like paws right up on the front of my body. I take a step back to brace myself.

"Get down, Gus!" Ms. Romero says. "I am so sorry. He is typically much better behaved than this. He's an agility and obedience trial dog. He knows not to jump."

"No worries, Ms. Romero. It's all part of the job," I say with a smile. "How is Gus doing at home?"

"Oh, he's just fine."

"How is his appetite, has he lost any weight?"

"Nope, none."

"Is he lethargic at home?"

"Goodness, no, he runs around constantly. I have to work to keep up with him."

"Is he drinking more water than normal? Do you have to fill up his water bowl more frequently?"

"Not really."

"Is there a new lump or swelling that you've noticed?" I ask while searching the pet parent's face.

"No, can't say I've noticed anything at all."

Hmm, this is not making sense. Does she know she booked an appointment with a cancer specialist? Before beginning a physical exam on the golden, I try one more time.

"What prompted you to come to see me?"

"Oh, well, a psychic told me to."

"A psychic?!"

"Yeah, an animal psychic. I was having a reading for Gus, and she said that he has cancer. My husband thinks I'm a nut, but I am worried sick. So, I made the first available appointment and here we are. I hope she is wrong, but I know deep down that she is probably right."

With that, I go to the ground to perform a physical exam. Gus is so excited he practically knocks me down. Ms. Romero helps to calm him. Carefully I palpate his body, listen to his heart and lungs. Unfortunately, the retriever has enlarged lymph nodes; my suspicion, as well as the psychic's, is that Gus has cancer, likely lymphoma. After I tell Ms. Romero of my concerns, she sits down and shakes her head.

"I knew it, I just knew it," the pet parent conceded. "The psychic was right."

Ms. Romero elects to have the necessary tests performed, and eventually Gus is treated with chemotherapy and goes into a complete remission. However, that day, as she hands me Gus's leash for the first time, she also places a calling card for the medium into my palm.

Rounding the bend to the technician station, I hand Gus off to my team with a list of instructions. I fill my techs in about the psychic and why Ms. Romero came to see us. Some look amazed; others look bewildered.

"You know, do you mind if I make a copy of that psychic's card?" Jackie asks, after the team has gone down the hall to the X-ray room with Gus.

"Sure, why, do you want to have a reading for one of your pets?" I inquire.

"No, Amanda, the tech in ICU, has been seriously worried. Her sister, who lives in Philadelphia, lost her orange tabby over a month ago. They can't find him anywhere. She's always talking about that cat. Maybe this psychic lady can help her."

"You know, that's a great idea. It certainly couldn't hurt to try."

A week later Amanda, the ICU tech, comes up to me while I am typing up my charts.

"Excuse me, Doc? Um, I wanted to thank you for your help."

"Sure, but how did I help?" I ask, perplexed.

"The phone number you gave us. That dog psychic. My sister had a session with her. The medium said that my sister's cat is safe. She said a little old lady took her in and was feeding her. While the psychic couldn't tell us where the cat was, she did describe exactly what the front door looked like. My sister and her boyfriend searched and searched throughout their neighborhood in Philly. And you're never gonna believe this: they found the door matching the description, and Cinnamon was there! It was amazing!"

"Oh, my goodness, that is so wonderful. I am so glad! My gosh, Ms. Romero did not steer us wrong."

I contemplate this happy news. Despite all my years of veterinary training, all the continuing ed meetings, trying to treat a case rationally and with eyes wide open, sometimes it takes a different approach to find an answer. At least that is the case for Gus and Cinnamon.

Back in my office, I think about another case that would not have such a happy resolution. But even here, I'd still been able to provide some comfort. Max was a small, fluffy, wheat-colored mixed-breed dog with a very large mass in his mouth. You could see the growth when he panted; you could also smell the stench a room away. The dog couldn't eat dry kibble anymore, though he was okay with canned dog food. Max's people had declined a biopsy recommended by their regular veterinarian, but they had allowed the vet to take two chest X-rays. Sadly, there were multiple nodules in the dog's lungs. The outlook was grim, but the couple still wanted to come in to speak with me. It turns out, they first noticed the mass six months ago, but they didn't take Max into the vet then because they didn't have the money. Week by week, the mass grew larger. They'd declined the biopsy because of the same financial straits—the husband had been out of work for months; the wife was pregnant. And now they were beating themselves up, feeling that they were at fault for Max's progressive cancer. The mass was darkly pigmented, likely melanoma. I told them that even if they'd come in right away when they first saw it, we couldn't have cured it. And that even if they won the lottery and had all the money in the world, we'd still be in the same place we are today. So, while I couldn't change the outcome, I could assure them that they were not in any way at fault or to be blamed. We discussed ways to make Max feel more comfortable at home for his last few weeks. It was a sad conversation, but at least when the couple left, the weight of guilt had been lifted off their shoulders.

117

At 4:00 p.m. the receptionist poked her head in, getting me out of my little reverie.

"Excuse, me, Doc, do you want me to put your last case in your room? They just arrived."

"Thanks, I can do it. I'll be right out."

I pick up the chart for Bogart, a ten-year-old yellow labradoodle with a history of allergies, the occasional hot spot, and foreign-body removal surgery (this pup has a taste for socks). He's been on arthritis medication for years, though over the past few months, the pain when he walks has increased. The family has come in for a second opinion, just to make sure they leave no stone unturned. They noticed a mass over his shoulder, which was deemed inoperable due to its large size. The dog has also lost weight. I tell my team that if they need me, I will be in the appointment. Cassidy does a few steps from the hip hop video "Cupid Shuffle." I smile and keep walking.

I meet the Porters in the waiting room: dad, mom, daughter, and son. Clearly, Bogart is a beloved member of the clan. The parents stand up to greet me while the kids keep texting on their cell phones. But Bogart just lies there, wagging his tail but not getting up. I introduce myself and lead the family into an exam room. The dad lifts Bogart's back end, which helps to kick-start him walking. Even so, he ambulates slowly and is a bit ataxic, walking as if he were drunk. It's sad to watch as Bogart trails behind his people.

In the exam room, I get on the floor to perform a physical.

I feel a bit self-conscious with the whole family watching me on the ground—this would have been a good day not to have worn a dress. But being a big dog, Bogart is much more comfortable on the floor than he would be on the exam table. And with his motor issues, it would be a lot to ask for him to come up to my eye level. Bogart doesn't seem to mind my manipulating the mass on his shoulder, so I can assume it's not painful. However, when I palpate down his spinal cord, he flinches in discomfort. This isn't adding up. The labradoodle's heart and lungs sound fine, though his liver feels a bit enlarged. I get up off the floor, then wash my hands.

"I think Bogart has more going on here than just the mass," I say, treading carefully with kids in the room. "A mass, even a large one like the one on his shoulder, should not cause your dog to walk like he's walking. I know it's easy to think that this is all from this mass and his arthritis, but I'd like to do some tests."

"What do you think this is, Doc?" the dad asks me. I make a quick glance to their children to signal that this could be a delicate subject.

"Well, it could be a neurologic issue," I reply. "It could be spread from the reason that you came in to see me, but it could be something else. We'd need to do a full workup to find out. If you decide not to do this, I can certainly put him on some anti-inflammatory medication and some pain medication to try to help him feel better."

"That's what we did with our first dog. We never found out why he wasn't well, and I've never forgiven myself," Mrs. Porter admits. "Bogart is family, and we're fortunate that we're able to do whatever's needed for him."

Practicing veterinary medicine is a bit like detective work. Our patients can't tell us what's wrong, so we have to go on a systematic hunt. A good sleuth looks at each bit of information received, then adjusts the investigation with tests, all in the hopes of reaching a conclusion, or in this case, a diagnosis. Because Bogart will need a battery of tests, the Porter family elects to leave him with my service. We'll begin with X-rays of his chest, blood work, a urinalysis, an abdominal ultrasound, and an aspirate of the mass in question. I have their permission to do further tests, as needed.

Mr. Porter helps Bogart to a standing position. He hands me his leash, but just as the dog and I are to head out the door to begin the workup, both kids spring from their seats and put their arms around the doodle's neck. Mrs. Porter gives me a look, mom to mom, as if to say, "Please help our family." I walk over and give her a hug.

It isn't easy when our beloved pets have cancer. It is that much harder when children are in the mix. I remember when I first told Peter about the *C* word diagnosis I'd been given. The moment my son and I sat down on the sofa, I could tell he knew the topic was serious. I turned to face him, thinking, Oh God, give me the strength I need for this conversation. He looked at me with his sweet brown eyes, searching my face for some clue as to what this was all about. Putting my hand on his hand, I told him gently that I had the C word, and that I was to have surgery. Though my voice did not waver, it did get awfully quiet. I felt my heart drop, my son looked so worried. He just stared at me, not saying a word.

I told him that I would have a recovery period of about six weeks. Both chemotherapy and radiation therapy would still be options. The doctors were hopeful I wouldn't need them, but we'd have to await the pathology results to know. Peter looked at me, eyes not moving, and in response, I couldn't take my eyes off of him. He's my boy, my son. Even though his concern and uncertainty with the situation were palpable, he remained stoic. I wanted to burst into a screaming fit of tears.

"And it's okay to tell your friends," I added. "In fact, I think you should. Your friends come over and I might look different. And it can help to open up to them when you want to talk. Of course, your dad and I are always here, whenever you need us."

"But, Mom, you'll be okay, right? Everything will be fine, right?"

I closed my eyes. Please, Lord, help me to beat this, help me to stay in my son's life for many, many decades, I thought. Please. I opened my eyes as I answered.

"Well, they say my prognosis is good, and you know your mom, I am relentlessly persistent. Maybe even annoyingly so." A pencil-thin smile crossed my face. Peter smiled back. I tried to stay as strong as I could, but as we embraced the tears trickled out. He held on for a very long time.

In my oncology area, I brief my team on what we need to do for Bogart. They'll begin the tests, though first I'll perform the aspirate of the shoulder mass. He lies on the table as still as can be. Whatever is going on is affecting him significantly. After taking a few samples from the large lump, I head to the lab to stain the slides. Once the slides are prepared and dry, I take a look at them under the microscope. This mass is not the cause of Bogart's problems. This is a lipoma, or benign fatty accumulation. The hunt continues.

While Bogart's tests are being run, I begin my next appointment. This is a recheck for Mia, a six-year-old female Chihuahua. Mia had surgery two weeks ago to remove a mammary gland tumor. At the time of surgery, she was also spayed.

"How's Mia doing since surgery?" I ask her pet parent, Ms. Garcia.

"She seems fine. She's running and jumping. When can I take her cone off?" the woman asks.

"Well, let me look at her incision and I'll let you know." With that, I take the dog from Ms. Garcia's lap and place her on the exam table. Mia is sporting a red knit sweater, which I remove. Her incision is clean and intact, and the skin has healed.

"She looks good," I say. "We can take out her stitches to-day, and as long as she doesn't lick this area, she can have her e-collar off. We did get the biopsy back, and Mia is a very lucky girl—her tumor is benign." I see Ms. Garcia's eyes moisten with happy tears, which she dabs at with a tissue.

"So, she doesn't have cancer?"

"Correct, thank goodness. But I do recommend that we keep a close watch on her. Because she was spayed later in life, she has a twenty-six percent chance of developing mammary cancer. For female dogs that are spayed as puppies, before their first heat, there's only a point-eight percent chance of getting this type of cancer." I try not to be preachy; I'm just relying information. But unless a female dog is a show dog or has an underlying condition, neutering is often the better option for a whole variety of reasons.

Ms. Garcia thanks me profusely. She will keep a watch on Mia, then return in three months for a checkup. She puts the Chihuahua back in her sweater and carries her out of the room. I look down to notice that I have a hand on my lab coat in the area of my abdomen. Gently my right palm rests atop my own surgical area, similar to Mia's. I shake my head quickly, remove my hand, then step out of the exam room to follow up with Bogart's case.

I find the doodle's blood work on my desk. Most of the values are normal, though he has an elevation in his protein level, also known as his globulins. He also has an elevation in his calcium, and his kidney enzymes are up just a bit. The two most likely diagnoses so far would be kidney disease or cancer. Jackie hands me Bogart's urinalysis and tells me that his X-rays are completed. The urinalysis is normal. Bogart is able to concentrate his urine well, so kidney disease is likely off the list. The three most common cancers that can present this way are lymphoma, an anal gland tumor, and multiple myeloma—a disease originating in the bone marrow. On rectal palpation, Bogart's anal glands are normal, which should narrow the list of likely suspects to lymphoma and myeloma.

The dog's X-rays show that his lungs are clear—no masses, no fluid. I look to his ribs and the bones of his spine, which are visible in the three images from radiology. After a few minutes' inspection I notice that, along with arthritis, there are very small, circular lesions in these bones that should not be there. I point these out to Jackie, who is always interested in learning more about the science of animal care. These areas of bone damage are common in multiple myeloma, and they can be painful. This is most likely why Bogart had discomfort when I put the slightest pressure on his spine during his physical examination.

Multiple myeloma is a disease of the plasma cell. Plasma cells are normal white blood cells in our bodies. Though the cancer starts in the bone marrow, it can quickly spread to the liver, spleen, lymph nodes, and bones. It can cause the problems we're seeing with the doodle's blood work. I ask our internist to do an ultrasound, and I request that he take samples of Bogart's liver and spleen. To complete this workup, I then ask my team to take abdominal X-rays to inspect Bogart's lumbar spine and hip region. The images show more circular lesions in these bones, and that Bogart has hip dysplasia.

All four members of the Porter family come back to retrieve Bogart at 6:30 p.m., and they are eager to hear the news. I carefully tell them of my findings so far, and I explain that we'll have to wait for the results of the splenic and liver samples.

"So, he does have cancer, but maybe not what we thought?" Mr. Porter asks.

"That's what it's looking like, so far," I say. "And I'm very sorry." I pause, feeling the intense gaze of four sets of eyes. "We should know tomorrow, once I get the final pathology report. I'll call you with the results to discuss treatment options then. For now, I'm going to send him home with some pain medication."

I receive a chorus of thanks. Mr. Porter takes Bogart's leash to lead him out, and sadly, our patient walks like a very old fellow. His family trails slowly behind him, not wanting to rush their ailing dog. Mrs. Porter stays back for a moment to tell me how much Bogart means to all of them. She's hoping beyond hope that their dog will get one more summer to swim at the shore with her children. She seems to have more she'd like to add to his story, but she simply pauses, then thanks me again for my help.

The following day, my team and I drag in, tired from the previous day's appointments. It's only 9:00 a.m. but we're already discussing what to order for lunch. Food is a big motivator for us. I guess we're more like our patients than we realize! We settle on pierogies—not a typical office order, though fast becoming our go-to staple. Combined with music, the occasional treat of ordering lunch is a morale booster. It gives us something to look forward to. Shifting my thoughts back to work, I sift through the faxes that came in through the night. Bogart's aspiration cytology results are in this stack. The report confirms my suspicions. I call the Porters.

"Hi, Mrs. Porter, how are you?" I ask.

"Oh, Doctor, fine. Thank you. Let me get my husband so we can both be on the call," she says. I hear footsteps across a hardwood floor, then the sound becomes a bit muffled. "Hi, we're both here."

"Okay, great," I begin. "I was trying to be careful yesterday when your kids were present, but the tests now confirm that Bogart has a type of cancer called multiple myeloma." I explain the basic parameters of this disease. "Ideally we should do a bone marrow aspirate to fully complete the workup. As for the cancer, we can't cure it, but we can treat it. The cancer is what's giving him pain and trouble walking. His arthritis and hip dysplasia don't help the situation, but there's a good chance that, with chemotherapy pills, he'll improve and feel better."

"Pills? You mean we'll give them to him at home?" Mr. Porter seems confused.

"Yes, it will be two different pills, each given once a day. I'll need to see him back in two weeks, but then he'll need to recheck only once a month for blood work and a physical exam."

"Will they make him sick?" Mrs. Porter asks.

"With the chemotherapy pill, there's an eighty-five percent chance that he'll have no side effects. There's a fifteen percent chance of stomach upset. If this happens, it'll begin within the first four days. The second pill is prednisone, a steroid. With this drug he'll be hungrier, drink more water, urinate more, and have increased panting. At first those side effects will be more noticeable, but over the months, we'll decrease the dose and the side effects will diminish. However, while most dogs don't lose their fur with chemotherapy, the doodle part of him will." I then explain how a poodle's fur growth is similar to a human's hair. It's the poodle (doodle) that's given Bogart his soft, blond fleece-like coat. "He won't be bald," I go on, "but his coat will be rather sparse on his body, and he could lose the fur around his face—as if you'd shaved his muzzle. It depends how much poodle he has in him, compared to how much Labrador. Again," I add, "I'm so very sorry."

"We don't care what he looks like," Mrs. Porter assures me. "We just want Bogart to be around. So when can we begin? We don't want to do the bone marrow test. We would just like to start his treatment."

"Cassidy can have the medications ready for you to pick up at our front desk in a couple of hours. We're open twenty-four seven, so you can get them whenever is convenient. Until I see him again, please continue with his pain medication as well."

Driving home, I think about the Porters' unconditional love for Bogart. They'll feel the same way about him, fur or no fur. And here I sit, emotionally tortured over my hair thinned from chemo. Maybe I should try this unconditional love thing for myself, especially when vanity is so much work!

I'm grateful that I looked into a scalp cooling technique, specifically the Paxman cold cap, which has a chance of saving some of your hair when you're undergoing chemotherapy. I investigated it on the internet, then had to push a bit at the cancer center to get a prescription. I'm not sure they see the point. Becoming bald is the norm for so many of their patients, and, after all, hair will grow back. But this is my battle, not theirs.

Basically, the Paxman scalp cooling unit is a funny-looking swimming cap hooked to a machine that produces ice crystals on your head. This cooling limits blood flow to your scalp, thus limiting drug exposure to your hair follicles. For some people, it works very well, saving much of their hair. For other people, it doesn't do much. And of course, it isn't covered by my insurance. But since when did having to fork over a credit card stop me? I plan to try the cold cap at tomorrow's treatment. I wish I'd had this from the beginning, but better late than never.

In my room at the cancer center, whichever girlfriend who's driven me in assists me with putting on the cap. It's not easy, definitely a two-person job—like trying to put on a wet suit for your head, only one size too small. But I'm not in this battle for comfort. As the cap begins to cool (aka freeze), the tingling on my head reminds me of junior high in the Midwest, when we'd stand at the bus stop in the morning with wet hair. Why take the time to blow-dry when the temperature is ten below zero? In the winter months, our hair would freeze as soon as we left the house. When you touched it, it literally felt and sounded crunchy.

Some people warn that the cold cap is very uncomfortable; apparently, some women need antianxiety medication to wear it, and some can't take it and simply give up. Me? It was *nothing*! Yes, it was cold, but nothing like those winter mornings waiting for the bus. The worst part is the chin strap, so tight it makes it difficult to speak clearly or to eat. For eight hours. I'm sorry that I'm such lousy company for my girlfriend. But then I decide to take this a step further.

Aside from possible hair loss, some chemotherapy may also cause a peripheral neuropathy—where your fingers and feet go numb—which in some cases can become a lifelong issue. Knowing that this damage can make it difficult to button a shirt or tie shoelaces, or make you trip when you walk, I decide to take the matter of my fingers into my own hands. In doing my job, I need to be able to give intravenous injections to patients, who for me are sometimes dehydrated four-pound animals. Working with such a small target requires good fine motor function, not pins and needles in my fingers. So, in addition to the shower cap from *Frozen* on my head, I choose to sit here during chemo with ice packs wrapped around my hands and feet for the entire, eight-hour ordeal. I'm hoping that by limiting the blood flow to these little extremities, the chemotherapy will be limited and hence the side effects will be, too. But I am one cold sight to see!

Two weeks go by, and the Porters are due in. As I enter the exam room, their boy holds up pictures that he and his sister have drawn for me. In a rainbow of crayon colors, they've written a big "Thank You" on the top of each piece of art-work.

This time, Bogart stands up on his own, no strap, no assist from his dad. He walks over to me, tail wagging. He has a very subtle alteration to his gait, but overall, he's moving substantially better, no longer walking like an ancient dog. I rub his head and smile.

"Well, Doc, you did it. Bogart is back to his usual self," Mr. Porter begins.

"Yeah, he tried to eat one of my socks!" interrupts their daughter. Her mom casts the girl a look, as if to say, "Don't get too carried away." But it makes us all feel good that Bogart is well enough to want to eat a smelly sock.

I get down on the floor with the labradoodle. He still has most of his fur, and his tail is wagging so vigorously that it hits me on the back—thump, thump, thump—the entire time I'm attempting to evaluate him. I press lightly along his spinal cord and onto his hips. Bogart doesn't seem to notice or care—he just continues to wag away. I press a bit more firmly, putting some muscle into it this time, and still the dog seems not to mind—a very good sign. His hips are weak, but this is attributable to his arthritis and hip dysplasia. To fully assess the medication's effects, though, we'll need to run some blood work.

I take him to the back, and, once up on the table, Bogart has no interest in sitting still. His tail continues to wag, making a thumping sound on the stainless-steel surface, keeping the beat to the country music playing in the background. It's amazing how relief of pain and—we hope—reduction of his cancer can make a patient feel so much more energetic. Bogart is an eager, happy, wiggly doodle, which makes it a challenge to draw his blood. Perhaps he would benefit from a calming meditation tape like I listen to during chemo. When we're done, I help the dog down from the table. He leaves a few blond strands of fur as he walks away.

Leading him back to the waiting area, I catch my reflection in a window, and yes, I still have my hair. I know it's thinner, though everyone says it looks the same. I'm not supposed to put any product in it, blow it dry, use warm water, or really style it, which certainly doesn't help "the look." My son, Peter, now spends more time on personal grooming than I do. But, as long as my hair stays on my head, it's all good.

Returning to the exam room, I greet the Porters with, "I have good news—Bogart's protein level and calcium are coming down! His kidney enzymes are now normal."

Mr. Porter asks, "When can we expect the other values to get back to normal?"

"That will take time, possibly over the next couple of months. But they've definitely improved. I'm going to make some adjustments to his chemo dose, and I don't need to see him back for a whole month."

"That's wonderful," Mrs. Porter says. "Thank you so much.

We plan to take him to our shore home. Is that okay? Can he get in the water?"

"Absolutely. Let him guide you as to whether or not he wants to go in and for how long. But it's all about quality of life. You should also notice that each month, he'll become a bit stronger, have a bit more stamina."

"So, what are we looking at?" Mr. Porter asks. "What's his prognosis?" He's rather blunt, despite the fact that there are young ears possibly listening. Both kids are on their phones, but I'm cautious, nonetheless.

"Well, the average disease-free time is about a year and a half," I offer.

"So, he'd live to a nice ripe age," says the father. "Did you hear that, Bogart? You'll be an old man." Mr. Porter rubs the dog vigorously. Then the Porters gather their items to leave. Once again, Mrs. Porter stays back to speak with me privately.

"Truly, thank you for everything you've done for our Bogart," she begins. "My husband went through a terrible health scare with his mom years ago, and I got Bogart for him as a puppy, to try to cheer him up. He was so depressed. But it worked. I became so worried when Bogart got sick. It's been a very trying time, and Bogart reminds my husband of his mother. But I just worry that his sadness could come back if we lost our dog."

"I understand. It isn't easy. We all rely on our animals for so many different things. You're doing everything possible for

Bogart and for the rest of your family." I reach out and give Mrs. Porter a hug. "They're all very fortunate to have you," I say, as she opens the door to leave. "Have a wonderful time at the shore."

Bogart ends up being able to spend three more full summers at the ocean. He sees the children grow; he rides in the cart alongside Mr. Porter when he plays golf. Not only does the family keep in touch, letting me know how their dog is doing, but Mrs. Porter—Jill—and I become good friends.

Then one morning, I get a call. Jill thinks that Bogart's cancer is back. I tell her to bring him in. Walking into the exam room, I find the whole family. Their son now is taller than I am. Bogart still wags his tail, but slowly, and he makes no effort to rise. I see the drawn and worried looks on their faces. I immediately go down on the ground to greet the dog.

"Hi, sweetheart. You don't feel so well, do you," I say softly, stroking his head. The dog looks up at me with his brown flecked eyes. "Let's see what's going on."

I begin my systematic evaluation of his body. His heart and lungs sound just fine. All his lymph nodes are of normal size. His liver and spleen palpate normally. His eyes are clear. Despite some tartar, his mouth is unremarkable. The lipoma on his shoulder has changed very little in the three years that have passed. I press lightly all the way down his spine—no reaction—so I press a little more firmly. Still, surprisingly, no reaction. I give it more muscle, but still the dog does not flinch. I suggest that we begin with some screening blood work and X-rays, and the Porters agree.

Within fifteen minutes, I have Bogart's blood work back. Oddly, it's fine. His protein level is normal, as is his serum calcium. Bogart's kidney function is also good, especially for a thirteen-year-old labradoodle. I log on to the computer program to view his X-rays. Try as I might, I cannot find any lytic lesions in his vertebral (spinal) bones or ribs, or in any of his other bones. But I do see something that needs to be addressed. First, I page our orthopedist to confirm my suspicions. He comes in, reviews the X-ray images, and examines Bogart. We agree on the same, unfortunate diagnosis.

I go back to the waiting family, who look at me anxiously. They can tell that I don't have good news.

"What is it?" Mr. Porter blurts out. "Is it his cancer?"

"No, actually, his cancer is still in a remission." They seem puzzled. "It's not his cancer. Thankfully, that hasn't come back. It's his arthritis."

Mr. Porter grapples with this surprising twist. "Arthritis? Not cancer?"

"Correct. Unfortunately, his arthritis and hip dysplasia have gotten substantially worse. He can no longer compensate with the medications that he's on. I've consulted with our orthopedist, and we could try some other medications, but they may not help. Sometimes, acupuncture can provide some relief, but right now, I'm not optimistic about his prognosis." I look to the family—my friends—with loving concern.

"So he beat the cancer . . . but his arthritis is his problem . . ." Mr. Porter is still processing. "Well, I don't want to lose my dog, but I'd say that's a win."

His wife and I exchange glances. She doesn't see the silver lining that her husband does.

The family elects to try Bogart on some new medications. Both kids have their heads hung low. Mr. Porter uses a sling to help Bogart walk, and I watch as they leave. Jill puts her sunglasses on, trying her best to hide her red, moist eyes. My heart goes out to all of them. I'll call Jill tonight to see how they're doing.

A week goes by, and Bogart does not improve. I have a long phone conversation with the Porters about quality of life and what that means for their family dog. He's having more difficulty just getting up and walking, causing him to hold in his urine. At times, this leaks out where Bogart lies, but he doesn't seem to realize it. Jill doesn't mind washing his dog beds frequently, but this is not a good life for a labradoodle. I mention that sometimes, it's an old-age issue like this, rather than disease per se, that becomes the defining problem for a pet.

"You've done everything possible for Bogart," I tell her. "And as hard as this decision is right now, you've given him three more years to run on the beach, be with your family, spend more time in the golf cart. You've given him a wonderful life, and he's very fortunate to be a member of your family."

"I know," Jill says. Then she sighs. "It's just hard. I dread talking to the kids about it, but I know they must see this coming. No one wants Bogart to be uncomfortable."

"Let me know if you need any help talking to the kids. It is a hard conversation to have," I offer.

The couple elects to have a peaceful, at-home euthanasia for their beloved dog. They will hold a family meeting to talk to the kids about end-of-life options. I give them the name of a wonderful veterinarian whose mobile practice is limited to at-home euthanasia and hospice care.

"You have no idea how much you've given us over these years," Jill begins. "You've made our lives better by making our dog better. We can never thank you enough."

I thank her in return for the kind words. But truly, the pleasure is all mine. I only wish our pets could be with us longer.

7

SASHA

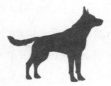

STAT call, line five, STAT call, bleeding abdomen," the receptionist shouts over the intercom. I rush to the phone.

On the other end of the line I hear, "Thanks for taking my
call. This is Dr. Smith. One of my patients was brought in a
few minutes ago. The dog's become acutely lethargic, no energy at all. His belly's distended, and when I put a needle into
his abdomen it came back with pure blood."

"Okay, send him right over," I say. "How long until he gets
here?"

"The family will leave right now. Maybe twenty minutes."

I hang up and I tell my team to prepare for an internal
bleeding emergency. Cassidy gets a gurney ready, while Jackie
collects a fluid bag, catheter, and intravenous medications

and sets up for a blood typing in case the dog needs a transfusion. The front desk is on the alert for their arrival.

"Gurney to the parking lot, STAT!" we hear over the intercom. The family must have flown.

My team responds accordingly. Two technicians steer the gurney down the ramp to the parking area. The pet parents have the hatch of their black Cadillac SUV opened up, their German shepherd lying on her side, panting heavily. The technicians greet the dog and then, on the count of three, lift her onto the gurney. Thankfully, she is small for a shepherd, not too heavy to lift. I ask the owners if it's okay for us to try to stabilize the dog, and they nod in unison. We quickly transport her to our treatment area.

The Vadamovas give the receptionist the necessary information as we wheel the dog to the back. Sasha is nine years old, spayed, with no past medical issues aside from a bout of Lyme disease some years ago, a right front leg injury when she was two, and a sensitive stomach. Her pet parents are extremely worried. Mrs. Vadamova sits down in the waiting room chair while her husband paces, nervously.

In the back, the dog is panting heavily and makes no attempt to get off the gurney as I look at her gums. They're white as can be, which tells me that she's very anemic. I listen to her chest, and her heart is racing—the body's response to blood loss. My team shaves a small area of brown fur from her right hind leg, then disinfects the site: first the blue Nolvasan scrub, then the alcohol. Jackie begins to place a catheter into Sasha's vein, but it collapses as she inserts the needle. The catheter won't feed—the tech can't get it in—but we need intravenous access to help stabilize and treat this patient. With blood loss, the shepherd's blood pressure is low, making her veins more difficult to work with. The technician will have to try another location, so we prep Sasha's left front leg, and the oncology nurse goes again. It takes a couple of tries, but this time, the catheter feeds smoothly. From this site, I have my team take blood samples so that we can better assess Sasha's condition. One nurse runs down the hall to the lab to perform the blood tests. She'll alert the internal medicine specialist that we need an abdominal ultrasound right away.

Just as we're hooking up IV fluids, the internal medicine veterinarian hurriedly pushes the ultrasound machine our way. He shaves Sasha's belly, then puts the cold blue ultrasound gel on the site. Sasha doesn't flinch—she must be in too much distress to care. The veterinarian moves the ultrasound probe methodically on her belly, then raises his brow, signaling that he's found the cause.

"She has a mass on her spleen that's bleeding into her abdomen."

"Any chance it's benign?" I ask, though we both know you can't tell based on an ultrasound alone.

"Not sure. But I'll look around to see if anything else is abnormal. Or if it's cancer, to make sure nothing's spread."

"Can you please check the heart, as well?"

"Already on it," he replies, as he begins a thorough evaluation.

I walk down the hall to see about the lab results, and my technician hands me the blood work. Yep, Sasha is anemic. Additionally, her clotting enzymes are a bit slower than we'd like. If the Vadamovas elect to proceed, Sasha will need extensive care.

As I round the corner and step into the waiting room, the couple get to their feet. They follow me into an exam room, a private place where we can have a difficult conversation.

"How is Sasha?" Mrs. Vadamova asks, her gray eyes frantically searching my face.

"She's hanging in there right now, and we're giving her fluids. Your veterinarian was correct, Sasha is bleeding into her abdomen."

Mrs. Vadamova puts her hand up to her mouth. Mr. Vadamova says nothing.

"She has a mass on her spleen, and that's the source of the bleeding."

"Is it cancer?"

"We don't know for sure. It could be. The only way to know for sure is with a biopsy. If you want, the next step would be for Sasha to have abdominal surgery to remove the spleen with the bleeding mass. Then we'd send this sample to the pathology lab to find out for sure. The odds are against us—

there's a greater chance this is malignant than not. If it's malignant, we can't cure her. But if it's benign, she'll be fine. The odds are about sixty-five to thirty-five malignant."

"I don't like those odds," Mr. Vadamova says.

"Me neither, but that's the truth," I tell him. "If you want to do surgery, she should have this done today by our surgical service. She'll need a blood transfusion first, and maybe another during or after the procedure. Sasha has lost a lot of blood, and her ability to clot is impaired."

I take a deep breath. "If you decide to not do the surgery—and there is no wrong answer here—you might then want to consider euthanasia."

This is never easy to say to pet parents. The Vadamovas say nothing, and their faces are blank. I step out of the room to give them time for all this to sink in. But not too much time—Sasha has very little to spare.

Moments later, Mr. Vadamova peeks his head out of the exam room door. "Hey, Doc?" he says. I step back into the exam room. The mood is somber.

"We've decided to do the surgery," he says. "To go all the way."

"You understand that if this is malignant, we can't cure her, right? If it is malignant, Sasha may still have a short prognosis, and there are risks with surgery. We'll stabilize her as best we can, but there's a chance she won't make it through the operation." A tear falls down Mrs. Vadamova's cheek. I put my hand on her shoulder.

"Doc, we gotta try," her husband says. "Where do I sign?"

Two technicians wheel Sasha into the elevator, which takes her to the second floor to be transferred to the surgical service. A blood transfusion has started, and she'll soon be prepped for the procedure. The surgical technicians will take chest X-rays first to make sure nothing has spread to the shepherd's lungs. Our surgeon is very skilled, and he's dealt with many critical cases like this one before. But still it's going to be touch and go. Assuming that Sasha makes it out of surgery, she'll stay on the service for days to receive care until she's strong enough to go home.

I head to my desk to complete Sasha's medical records, and I think about my own issues with bleeding. After my third round of chemotherapy, I developed a tennis-ball-sized swelling on my right arm, the one that had the IV catheter in it. The swelling was so sore that it would keep me awake at night. I decided to have it looked at so as not to delay my next chemotherapy treatment. My husband and I went to the cancer center, and it turned out I had a superficial blood clot. Thankfully, this required no real treatment aside from hot packs and home care. Unfortunately, however, with my next round of chemotherapy, I developed moderate phlebitis and many more clots on both hands and arms. Though these superficial clots were never a danger, they did scare me. More serious clots can break off and travel to places I didn't want them to go. My mind raced with unpleasant thoughts. When I'd fall asleep at night, I'd worry that I might not wake up.

At Sasha's two-week recheck, I enter the exam room to find a vastly different dog. The shepherd is circling the room, panting, full of nervous energy. She immediately comes up to greet me, wanting to be petted. I reach down and scratch her under her chin. As she looks up at me, her color is good, nice and pink. The Vadamovas are very different as well—at ease, sitting in the exam room chairs, smiling.

"She's back to our normal Sasha," Mrs. Vadamova says.

"I'm so glad," I respond, though I'm still a little tentative in my words. I take a brief history: Sasha has a good appetite, she has a normal activity level at home, and she's had no vomiting or diarrhea. Because she's a large-breed dog, I bend down to do a physical exam on the floor.

Sasha is very wiggly, thinking it's play time, so I ask a technician to come and help hold her. Sasha exhibits no signs of having had surgery, except for the missing brown and black fur that was shaved from her abdomen. Her sutures are still in place. Fourteen days after my abdominal procedure, I know I could never have gotten on the floor to play. It took many weeks to regain my normal gait and to stand up straight.

Despite all these positive signs, once back on my feet, I have to say, "Unfortunately, I don't have good news." The couple look at me anxiously.

"According to the pathology report, Sasha has a very aggressive type of cancer called hemangiosarcoma. It is the most common tumor that occurs in the spleen of a dog. It arises from the lining of blood vessels, which gives it instant access to the bloodstream. Which means that this type of cancer can spread very quickly." The faces of the Vadamovas fall. "I'm so sorry," I say.

"What can we do, Doc?" Mr. Vadamova asks.

"Well, you've already helped her a great deal by having the surgery. You gave Sasha back her quality of life." Obviously, I'm trying to look on the bright side. "Unfortunately, with surgery alone, her prognosis is typically only three months."

"Three months!" the man shouts.

"Yes. I really am sorry," I answer. "We could try chemotherapy. In general, dogs do well with chemotherapy." I go through my repertoire about this modality, the side effects, the schedule, and the costs.

Mr. Vadamova appears angry. "So, we can't cure her?"

"No, we can't," I carefully reply, brushing past his tone. Mr. Vadamova slams his fist on the counter. I jerk back, and his wife stares at the ground. "But there's a chance chemotherapy can help. Typically . . ." I'm treading lightly here, trying not to raise unrealistic hopes. "Typically it can help for about six months. About ten percent of dogs will be in a remission for

146

one year. But we need to remember that these are averages. Some dogs don't do as well; some dogs do better. Right now, we have to assume that Sasha is the average dog." The Vadamovas say nothing. They just look at me while the information whirls in their heads. "I will step out to give you some time to talk. If you decide to do chemotherapy, we could begin as soon as today. If you decide not to pursue chemotherapy, that's fine, too. There's no wrong answer here." I leave the couple and their dog in the exam room.

In a busy practice, it is easy to lose track of time, and I don't want to leave the Vadamovas in the room too long. Should they have any further questions, I want to be present. I give them ten minutes, then I knock softly on the door and reenter the room. Mrs. Vadamova has been crying. She blots her eyes carefully, trying to preserve her makeup.

"Do you have any other questions?" I ask.

"No. We want to treat," Mr. Vadamova says flatly, and then he hands me the dog's leash.

I take Sasha to the back. Or, more accurately, Sasha pulls me out the door and down the hall. Right now, she's strong and feels good. She greets my oncology trio as eagerly as she greeted me in the exam room. As the techs put the dog on the scale to weigh her, they have trouble keeping her still. But with quality of life being the goal here, too much energy is a good problem to have. I jot down her weight, then calculate her chemotherapy dose. Jackie draws up the medication in the biologic safety cabinet, wearing full PPE. The other two oncology nurses position Sasha on the treatment table, but she's still a wiggle worm. Not wanting to resort to sedation, we ask a third technician to step in, and with the extra pair of hands we manage to quiet the dog. We pet Sasha and tell her what a good girl she is. Given the dog's nice, healthy veins, the technician has no difficulty this time accessing her blood vessel to administer the chemotherapy. In ten minutes, Sasha is done and jumps off the table.

Cassidy brings Sasha back to her pet parents, who wait with open arms. We ask them to speak with Tiara at the front desk to make a recheck appointment for Sasha's next chemotherapy treatment three weeks from now. I finish up Sasha's chart and turn off my computer for the night. It's been a long day of cases, and I'm looking forward to getting home. As I hang up my lab coat, Tiara comes back, looking stunned.

"Everything okay?" I ask.

"It's just weird, that's all," she says.

"What's weird?"

"Mr. Vadamova. This is the second time he's made me call another client and move their appointment to a different slot."

"What? Why would he do that?"

"Because he wants a particular appointment, day and time. He won't settle for even thirty minutes later. I shouldn't have done it, but I did. He's very intimidating."

"Any other issues?"

"No, but he must be super rich. He pays in all cash. Even for Sasha's emergency surgery bill. I've never seen so much money all at once."

"Hmm. Well, Mr. Vadamova shouldn't tell you to move someone else's appointment. If we need to juggle things, I should be involved, but strong-arming you isn't appropriate. I'll speak with him when I see them next."

A few weeks later, I decide to get to the office a little early to catch up on some paperwork. I glance at my appointment schedule for the day and see that the Vadamovas are due in at 10:30. Weird that the man wanted a mid-morning appointment. Most people with busy schedules want to come in first thing or have the last appointment of the day.

Ten-thirty comes and ten-thirty goes. No Sasha. At 10:50 a.m., Tiara places a call to the Vadamovas' cell number, which goes straight to voice mail. There's no answer on their house line either, so the receptionist leaves a message. Ten minutes later, the Vadamovas' black Cadillac pulls up in the parking lot. They slowly walk Sasha on the grass to see if she needs to go, but she just sniffs. At 11:05 a.m. I walk outside in my lab coat to get this appointment started.

"Hi," I start out while walking through the parking lot to the grassed section. The Vadamovas turn to look at me. "We weren't sure you were coming. You've actually missed your appointment."

"You can just treat Sasha now," Mr. Vadamova tells me.

"Normally I would have an eleven o'clock appointment already booked, but we're lucky—today I don't. I would never turn Sasha away, though. If you miss your appointment, I am happy to fit you in. It's just if the next appointment comes on time, I will have to see them first and you would then have to wait."

"I don't want to wait," Mr. Vadamova tells me. Obviously, this is a man who typically gets what he wants.

"You don't have to wait today. But you might have, if I'd had an appointment booked. It's not fair to the other person who comes on time. Which brings me to another topic. If you need a certain time for your appointment that's unavailable, ask me. We can't have the receptionist move some other person's appointment." I'm looking directly into his eyes. He stares back at me sternly but says nothing. "Is there a reason you need a certain time? Maybe I can help."

"Nope. I just like ten-thirty," he admits. I continue to look him in the eye, until his face softens and he looks away. We all head into the building. With me needing to hold my ground like this, I am glad we ordered big sandwiches for lunch today.

I bring Sasha to the back for her blood to be drawn. She

continues to be her energetic self, an indication that she's doing well, and by now we know how to handle her. My team holds her still while I draw her blood, then perform a physical exam. I check her gums. Nice and pink. Sasha's heart rate is 120 beats per minute, right where it should be. The lungs are clear. Her abdomen palpates normally, no enlarged organs. I review her blood work; all looks good. Before giving her the second chemotherapy treatment, the oncology nurse pages for a third pair of hands. We can't have Sasha move during treatment, and, for her sake, we'd rather not sedate her. She is a happy girl and, as before, behaves with three people gently holding her as she lies on her side. Once chemotherapy has finished, the catheter's been removed, and the vein has clotted, the dog jumps off of the exam table. She then pulls my technician out the door to the waiting room, where she's welcomed by the Vadamovas' beaming smiles.

I see two more patients, and then it's time for lunch. On my way to the staff room, I stop to inquire at the reception desk.

"Tiara, were there any issues when the Vadamovas checked out?"

"No, I gave them an open slot for their next appointment. He still paid with a wad of cash. Maybe they have a son my age," she chuckles. I give her a friendly eye roll, then head up to eat my lunch.

The next time Sasha is scheduled, the family arrives right on time. The Vadamovas report that she's doing well, remaining active and keeping up her appetite. Sasha comes to the back, walking nicely with the nurse. She hops up on the table and the tech pushes the button to raise her up. Sasha is not so wiggly today, making it easier to draw her blood. On physical examination, I notice that while her gums are pink, they're less rosy than before. This could be nothing, but five minutes later, when I'm handed her blood work, I see that her red blood cell count has dropped—she's anemic. I need to let the family know.

I head to the waiting room and inform the Vadamovas that we need to talk in the privacy of an exam room. Mrs. Vadamova looks very concerned.

"So, Sasha is really fine at home? Not lethargic at all?" I look at each of their faces in turn.

"Well, I think she's quieter at home," Mrs. Vadamova now admits. "And she does sleep more."

"She's *fine*," Mr. Vadamova insists, as if to settle the matter. Then he turns to his wife and says, "You don't know."

"I *do* know," she says in defense. "I'm home with the dog all day."

I clear my throat, and swallow hard.

"Well, I don't have good news. Today, she's anemic. Which makes me think she would be quiet at home." I look kindly in Mrs. Vadamova's direction. "I'd like to do an abdominal ultrasound to see—"

"Yes," Mr. Vadamova cuts me off. "Do the test. We'll wait."

And with that, I go back to request the procedure.

The internist finishes up with a Jack Russell, retrieving a piece of wood that was stuck in his mouth—silly dog. When he's ready, my team leads Sasha to the Intensive Care Unit.

I sit down at the computer to update the dog's chart. About twenty minutes go by, and I'm getting impatient. I need to know what's going on with Sasha.

I go down to ICU, stick my head in, and say, "See anything?"

The internist is still moving the probe slowly back and forth on the dog's belly.

"Nothing good," he responds.

He and I confer for a few moments, then I prepare myself for telling the Vadamovas the bad news.

When I enter the waiting room, they both stand up in anticipation. My demeanor is enough to give them the gist. Quietly, they follow me into an exam room.

"What is it?" the husband asks.

"Her cancer has spread to her liver. It's—"

"Can we remove it?" Mr. Vadamova blurts out. "If it's a matter of money, we'll pay anything."

"Unfortunately, it's spread throughout the liver, in all her lobes. It's too extensive for surgery to do any good. I'm so sorry."

I pause to give them time to absorb. "And even if you had all of the money in the world," I continue, "it wouldn't change a thing right now for Sasha."

I sit down next to them and take Mrs. Vadamova's left hand. She pats my hand with her right, then lets it rest atop mine. We sit in silence.

"Her cancer is much more aggressive than the average dog's. You've done the best possible for her. We could try a different chemotherapy protocol, but I think it would be of very little benefit."

"I think we should just take her home," Mr. Vadamova offers. His wife nods, then stares at the floor. She grips my hand more tightly. "How . . . how will we know when it is time?" she asks.

"The most important thing is her quality of life. And she will have her own way of telling you. You know her so well. But as the cancer progresses, she'll begin to feel really lousy, like we do when we have the flu. The disease will compete with her body for energy, so she'll be much quieter at home." Mrs. Vadamova nods her head, acknowledging what she's already seeing during the day. "You might notice that Sasha begins to lose weight despite having a good appetite. This is because the cancer will utilize the nutrients that she eats. Eventually, her appetite may decrease. It's just like my husband. Normally he could eat a cheeseburger twice a day, every day, but when he has the flu, all he wants are crackers and maybe some Cup of Soup." I'm trying to lighten the mood.

"And, of course, Sasha could experience another bleed, like before. This would be a medical emergency. She may not come back from this if it happens. At that point, you may be faced with another decision."

"She won't be in pain?" Mr. Vadamova asks.

"No, thankfully she won't," I confirm.

The Vadamovas tell me they understand. They elect to take their girl home to enjoy the time she has left. The family realizes we may only be talking about weeks. I instruct them to call me with any questions, and I remind them that the hospital is staffed twenty-four hours a day, seven days a week, with emergency veterinarians if needed. Mrs. Vadamova expresses her appreciation and we hug. Sasha walks with Mrs. Vadamova to the parking lot as Mr. Vadamova goes to pay the bill.

The end of chemotherapy should be a celebratory occasion. Unfortunately, it is not that way in Sasha's case. Typically when one of my four-legged patients has completed chemotherapy, we make a big deal of it, for it is an accomplishment worth celebrating. My technicians and I, with ear-to-ear smiles, head to the waiting room, greeting the family with a personalized diploma and loving hugs. Sometimes we even snap a few photos. Moist eyes fill the room at this happy time. Occasionally, Jackie will play the theme song from *Rocky* on her cell phone as we walk toward the pet parents. Always good to know how to set a mood.

For me, I am now officially finished with my chemotherapy. Odd how anticlimactic it is. It's as if I received one last blow, one last sucker punch (though in IV chemotherapy form), and am now left having to hold myself in this space. I feel deflated, and yet I should feel elated. When I finished the radiation therapy treatments, there was a loud brass bell to ring and a waiting room full of patients and staff clapping. Today there is no bell, no congratulatory remarks. It is late in the day. The support staff are already cleaning this wing of the treatment center. A nurse is finishing paperwork at her desk. No one "sees" me. It is incredibly lonely. I gather my belongings, clutching them close to my chest as I slowly shuffle out of the large gray building; I am a worn-out shell. Dusk has settled in. All I want to do is go home and hide.

We get used to seeing the animals and their families week after week. I get very used to it. While it is wonderful that a pet has completed their protocol, there is a part of me that will miss seeing our four-legged friend, miss chatting with their family members. It is as if a part of myself has walked out the door when they leave.

For me personally, there is some security in being a patient, having your treatment team see you every few weeks, do blood work, make sure you are fine. I feel I am now sent out into the world to flounder. But I do know that my doctors will follow me closely, every three months in fact. My medical oncology team says this is the time that they start counting as my remission. Thank God all gross (i.e., macroscopic) disease was removed surgically. I went through all the chemo and radiation in the hope of obliterating any and all microscopic cancer cells. But now it is just a waiting game. Praying it doesn't come back, wondering as each week passes: Am I missing a sign? Could it be growing silently? Deep breaths. Reminding myself of the importance of believing it will be alright, the importance to be grateful for each day.

Two weeks later, I phone the Vadamovas to check up on Sasha. Mrs. Vadamova answers.

"Yes, yes, Sasha seems just fine. She does sleep more, but she's eating and going to the bathroom normally."

"Good. I'm glad to hear that. How's the color of her gums?" I ask. There is a pregnant pause.

"Hello?"

"I'm here. I don't want to look at her gums," the woman admits. "I don't want to know."

"Okay, no worries, you don't have to. I was only asking. It's all okay." I don't want her to feel worse than she already does. This process is different for all of us. "As long as Sasha has a good quality of life and enjoys being with you, that's what's most important." We both hang up. I make a note for myself to continue checking in with this family.

Another week goes by, and I again reach out. This time, Mr. Vadamova picks up.

"She's fine. Really, Doc, there's no problem. We'll call you if there's an issue." His tone is abrupt and cold.

"Okay, we're here if you need us." I hang up and throw away my yellow sticky note reminding me to call them. I pick up the next chart on the stack, ready to begin my next appointment.

The following week, no word from the Vadamovas. On the fifth week, Jackie calls Sasha's regular veterinarian to see if they've heard anything. They have not. On the sixth week, at the early hour of 7:00 a.m., just as I'm taking off my coat and logging into my computer, I see that someone has placed Sasha's chart on my workstation. Likely not a good sign. I throw my coat on the back of my chair and pick up the chart. I riffle through the pages and see that Sasha has been acutely lethargic at home. She might even have collapsed from profound weakness. The Vadamovas brought her into the ER here at 10:00 p.m. last night. She was terribly anemic, her gums white. Due to her deteriorated state and poor quality of life, the family elected a humane euthanasia.

Though the Vadamovas made the right decision, I'm sure it wasn't easy. It never is. Humanely ending an animal's life is something that can tear you up inside, but no matter how gut-wrenching, it can be the most selfless decision a pet parent can make. You don't want your beloved companion to suffer. And for the veterinarian, knowing that this procedure can be the right and sometimes necessary thing doesn't make it any easier to perform. I have to really concentrate to put the catheter into the vein and give the drugs, struggling to remain stoically professional while my eyes threaten to flood with tears. If I start crying, I won't be able to see what I am supposed to do. Even when I know that this is best for a dog or cat, it still makes me profoundly sad to see how much the pet parents suffer.

For some individuals, euthanizing their pet is either too hard for them to decide to do or a decision that conflicts with their belief system. It's important that they understand that there is no one right decision, and that the veterinarian's office is a judgment-free zone. Hospice care, medications given to improve an animal's comfort, also can be used during a patient's final days.

I reach for the phone to call the Vadamovas, then realize it's too early. When my team files in to begin our morning, I alert them of what's happened the night before. Jackie brushes a tear from her eye; Cassidy excuses herself to go to the bathroom—a classic move whenever she wants to cry alone. Jackie asks if I need a hug. I nod yes, and we hold each other for a moment, weeping.

At 9:00 a.m.—a respectable time to call, even if the family had a tough, late night—I dial the Vadamovas' number. The phone rings and rings, and finally, the answering machine picks up. I leave a message, offering my deepest sympathies and asking the family to call if they would like to speak. I set the phone down and feel empty.

At the end of our workday, we still haven't heard from the Vadamovas. The grieving process takes time, I understand all too well. We'll send a condolence card to the family, and we'll be here if they need us.

On Friday, I hang up my coat and head to my workstation at 6:50 a.m., ready to begin the last day of what's been a rough week. I need to focus on what's ahead, but I can't help thinking about the Vadamovas, wondering how they're coping with their loss.

Tiara comes back and interrupts my thought process. "Excuse me, you have a visitor," she says.

"A visitor? Who?" It's rare to have someone just show up, especially at 6:50 in the morning.

"It's Mr. Vadamova." The young receptionist's eyes are as

big as saucers. "He says he needs to speak to you privately in the exam room. He seems serious."

Hmm, that is strange. I hope he isn't angry again. I could understand Mrs. Vadamova wanting to talk, but not her husband.

"Okay, have him go to room two, I'll be there in a sec." I put my lab coat on and gather my thoughts.

When I enter the exam room, Mr. Vadamova is standing tall, holding his hat.

"Hi, I'm so sorry about Sasha," I begin. "She was such a good dog. And you did everything possible for her."

As I'm speaking, I'm still wondering why he's come in, and so early.

"Thank you," he says. "I had to pick up Sasha's ashes, and I wanted to speak with you."

I swallow hard. Speak about what? I heard him loud and clear weeks ago when he didn't want to talk. "Well, it is nice you came in. And again, I am so very sorry. I wish Sasha had had more time."

"My wife and I appreciate your help. Really. I want you to know that if you ever need anything, you can call me," Mr. Vadamova offers.

"Thank you."

"No, really, if you need anything, call me."

"Okay, thanks."

"Doc, let's just put it to you this way. If you ever need *any-*

thing, call me. If you ever need a favor, call me. If anyone is ever *bothering* you, call me. Understand?"

He says all this very emphatically, then adds a knowing wink.

Holy mackerel! Now it dawns on me. I go weak in the knees thinking how naive I'd been—laying down the law about making appointments and arriving on time. I could have survived blood clots, only to "sleep with the fishes" for being too bossy in a doctor-client relationship! And where is Tiara now in case I need her? My mind races. I hope she's keeping an eye on this exam room entrance.

Mr. Vadamova starts toward the door, then stops, turns, and pats my shoulder.

After he leaves, I collapse into a chair and call my husband.

"Hi, honey. You've heard me talk about Mr. Vadamova? You'll never guess what he does for a living."

I then tell Mike the whole story, with special emphasis on Mr. Vadamova's idea of a "thank-you" gift.

"And, honey," I say, "given my new friend, from now on, you'd better think twice before giving me any lip!"

8

FRANNY AND LUCKY

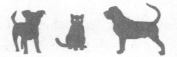

Autumn is upon us—my favorite season. My childhood in the Midwest was filled with yellow, red, and orange maple leaves, cider mills, and big cozy sweaters. On this weekday morning, like any other, I long to be outside, walking through the leaves, listening as they make a crunching sound with each step I take. But I am in my routine, driving my son to school. I'm not quite sure he is fully awake, but he is on time today, so we have to consider that a success.

I drop him off, and just after pulling out of the school's driveway, I get a call on my cell. The car monitor tells me it's Peter. Great, just as I was celebrating this small timeliness victory, my mind races: What did he forget now? He should be more organized! I don't have the time to rush back home to get whatever he needs, but I know I'll still do it. I keep my snarky thoughts to myself.

"Hey, hon, what's up?" I ask.

"Could, uh, could you come back for a second?" Peter stammers.

"What for?" I reply, quickly glancing in the back seat to see if he left something there. Wouldn't be the first time.

"Well, we need your help. Colin and I found a little cat that looks injured. Please, Mom?"

"Sure, I'll turn around," I say, then pull an illegal U-ie.

On reaching the school, I park my station wagon. I see a group of students huddled in a circle, and I have a hunch to head there. As I approach, the kids part, allowing me to enter their ring, where I find a disheveled gray cat that had clearly been out on the streets for a while.

"The cat was just lying here, meowing," Peter informs me. "I'm not sure it can walk."

I bend down and approach the animal cautiously. An injured animal can be unpredictable. Even the nicest animal can lash out when in pain. I reach over gently, slowly, and the kitty allows me to pet its head. I scratch a bit behind its right ear, and she (I am only assuming at this point) presses into me, a sure sign that she likes what I am doing. Carefully, I begin to examine the stray. Her coat is matted and full of burrs. She is skin and bones. But the biggest issue is that her left rear limb is limp. She tenses a bit as I touch the leg but is sweet and trusting. She does not try to bite.

"Okay, you guys, I think her leg is fractured, but with a little care, we might be able to fix her," I inform the teens. "She is really sweet."

The school bell rings abruptly, startling everyone.

While the other students scatter off to their classes, Peter stays with me.

"Go, sweetheart, I'll be okay," I say to my son.

"No, you'll need help getting her to the car. It's no big deal if I'm a few minutes late to first period. Besides, it wouldn't be the first time," he grimaces. "And I don't want to leave you alone with this," he admits.

I give him a look of "What am I going to do with you?" but down deep, I know my son has a good heart. Peter runs into the school and comes back with a box. I gingerly lift the cat up and place her in the cardboard container. She does not struggle but watches us intently. Peter carries the box as we walk to the car. He sneezes; poor kid is allergic to cats. I open the passenger side door and he places our new friend in her box on the front seat. Normally, I would not condone putting a pet in the front of a vehicle, but I want to keep a hand on the box and an eye on her.

"Hey, Peter, thank you. You did a good thing today," I say lovingly.

"Sure, Mom, no problem." He flashes me a smile, sneezes again, then runs back up to the school.

The drive to work is uneventful. I phone in to let my team know why I am a bit late, and that I'm bringing a new patient with me. I offer to buy them lunch, knowing that I'm adding to their workload. Two of my technicians greet me at the side door. They take the box, cooing over its contents.

"Be careful with her, she's a stray," I instruct, but they know how to handle a stray. "I need to do a full physical exam on her. But let me see my first appointment of the day. I feel bad for keeping them waiting. In the meantime, please run a full blood panel on her, and if all is okay, give her some sedation/pain medication to get some X-rays on that back leg. You should probably put a muzzle on her, just in case. And don't forget to pick a place for lunch."

The cat's blood work is completely normal. No kidney issues, no infectious diseases such as feline leukemia virus or feline immunodeficiency virus. That is good news. A review of her limb radiographs reveals a noncomminuted, simple fracture. In other words, she has a very clean break of her tibia, or shin bone, which should heal with supportive care alone.

"I'll have the orthopedic surgeon review her X-rays to confirm my diagnosis, and then they can place a splint on her. She is lucky that she doesn't need surgery," I tell my team. "But before you take her to them, and while she's still sedated, please carefully give her a bath, clip her nails, and clean her ears. She has clearly been roaming the streets for quite a while. After which, let's get an IV catheter in her for fluids and nourishment. Thank you."

Two technicians take her over to the bathing table while Cassidy and I treat a patient with chemotherapy. The soundtrack from *Pretty in Pink* plays on the background. Twenty minutes later, I look over at the team of two, wondering why the bath is taking so long. As I approach, I notice a complete change in the cat.

"Well, it looks like I was wrong, she's not a gray cat at all," I say in surprise. "I can't believe she's actually a *white* cat! Who knew!"

"Yeah, we kept washing and washing. Her color got lighter and lighter. And, um, no offense, but you were wrong a second time as well . . . She's a *he*!" We all chuckle a bit as I slowly shake my head and walk away.

With rehydration and good meals over a few days, Sultan, as we've named him, should lead a happy, healthy life. But Sultan can't stay with us for long. We're a hospital for the sick, and Sultan only needs strict rest, good groceries, and some tender loving care.

"We don't want to send Sultan to the shelter," my head tech informs me as the other two technicians stand behind her. I stop typing and look up from the computer.

"Neither do I. Don't worry, though, I have a plan," I reassure the team. I turn back to the computer, but instead of finishing the chart that I was working on, I look up an old client's phone number. I know the family has moved, but I hope their phone number has remained the same. I dial, fingers crossed that they are ready for a new addition.

"Hello?"

"Hi, Mrs. Robinson. Long time, no talk. I hope you and your family are well," I reply.

"Why, yes, we are, Doctor. It is so nice to hear your voice! We are so appreciative of all that you did for Clementine. You know, each Thanksgiving, you are on our list of people we are grateful for. We just can't thank you enough."

"That is very kind. I just wish Clementine could have had a bit longer," I admit.

"Oh, please, she was a crabby seventeen-year-old orange tabby. She lived a long life."

"I like crabby. Anyway, the reason that I am calling is, well, I was wondering, would you be interested in adopting a wonderful, stray cat that we recently found? In thinking of new homes for the cat, I thought of you first."

I proceed to tell Mrs. Robinson about Sultan and his needs for care. Intrigued, we set a time for her to visit the cat. I hang up the receiver, feeling rather assured that she will take him home. Sultan will have a good family to love him.

Duty calls, and I pick up the next chart to review before going into the appointment.

Franny is an eight-year-old, spayed, female bloodhound. Her history includes Lyme disease and lipomas, or benign fatty tumors. She's coming in today for a consult after having had surgery for a mass in her stomach.

"Good morning, Mr. . . . uh . . . Officer Nelson," I say, correcting myself mid-sentence as I take in the man's dark blue uniform. From the look of her harness, I have to assume that Franny is a member of the force as well. She's sitting by her partner's side, at attention, with a long string of drool hanging from her jowl.

I take Franny's history and learn that she's a search-and-rescue dog. She and Officer Nelson receive calls from all over the state to assist in finding missing people, as well as bad guys on the run. Franny is so good at her job—she's found lots of lost people—that she's become a celebrity with her own Facebook page.

The urgency in her care is not just that the police academy made a major investment in this bloodhound—raising her from a puppy and giving her extensive training. As so often happens, Officer Nelson has adopted Franny as part of his family. During her hours off-duty, Franny lives with the Nelsons and enjoys the comforts of their home.

I've consulted and cared for other working dogs. I've treated many Seeing Eye dogs who are afflicted with cancer, yet still eagerly guide their visually impaired person. With guide dogs, a veterinary oncologist has to strike the balance between extending the animal's life and risking the side effects of treatment. It takes years to raise a steady guide dog, and the animal really has to be on her game to keep the visually impaired individual out of harm's way. I've also treated bomb-sniffing dogs and drug-sniffing dogs, which has been known to create odd situations in the waiting room. One day, Officer Leroy and his German shepherd came in for a recheck appointment, and he overlapped with another client whom we suspected of being under the influence. When the client saw the K-9 team, he rushed into an empty exam room and slammed the door, trying to hide!

In general, Franny has been a healthy dog. Her past bout of Lyme disease isn't surprising, given all the woods and fields she traverses while tracking scents on the job. Her Lyme responded to a monthlong course of doxycycline, the antibiotic of choice for this tick-borne illness. Recently, though, Franny has been losing weight. First, she no longer finished all her food; then, she started vomiting. This is when Officer Nelson brought her into the internal medicine service for a workup. With ultrasound, the internist found a mass at her pylorus, one of the regions in her stomach. It was too large to remove via endoscopy, so Officer Nelson and his colleagues elected for Franny to undergo surgery. It's been three weeks since the procedure, and now here she is in front of me.

"How's Franny been doing since the operation?" I inquire.

"You know, she's much better. Her appetite is better, though not yet back to where it used to be."

"Has she had any more vomiting?"

"No, none. I'm still feeding her soft foods the way the surgeon recommended. And smaller, more frequent meals like I was told." Officer Nelson then takes a tissue and wipes the long drool from Franny's face. It's clear that this policeman has had to wipe many strands of drool from his partner's furry lips over the years, and, while this clearly is routine, likely something he "just does," the officer does it with great care. "When can she go back to her regular feedings? And can I work her now? She loves to work."

"It's been three weeks, so it's fine to go back to her normal food. But please remember to reintroduce it slowly—like over the next couple of weeks. She could have some GI upset if you move too fast."

The policeman nods.

"As far as working her goes, as long as she's up for it, it's fine to have her back in the field."

A big grin comes across his face, and he vigorously rubs Franny under her ear and chin.

Franny is too big to put up on the exam table, so once again, like a gymnast, I resort to the floor exercise. She's so tall, however, that I need only bend from the waist to listen to her heart and lungs with my stethoscope. I gently palpate her abdomen—it's soft and not painful—however, I need to be careful in this region due to her healing incision. I then hold Franny's head, looking at her face straight on. She looks back at me with droopy lids over chestnut-colored eyes. I lift up her jowls to examine her mouth. Boy, does this dog produce a lot of drool! I should have put on a pair of exam gloves. Lastly, I need to inspect the surgical site, which, given that it's on her belly, is when I need to get down on my hands and knees to look up and under. The incision is CDI—clean, dry, and intact. I stand up, straighten my dress—again, not the best wardrobe choice for crawling under larger dogs—as well as my lab coat, then wash and dry my hands.

"The type of cancer that was in Franny's stomach is called a mast cell tumor," I begin. "It's the most common skin tumor in a dog. We don't see it as often in the GI tract, but it can hap-

172

pen. It occurs more commonly in this area in the stomach or intestines in cats. Unfortunately, in this site in a dog, we can't cure it. From the biopsy report, we know that there are still some microscopic cancer cells that have been left behind."

I give the officer a sympathetic look. Telling unpleasant truths is the hardest part of my job.

"And, unfortunately, the prognosis isn't very good."

The policeman stares intently, hanging on my every word.

"It may be only a few months. But we can try to treat the disease with chemotherapy," I add, always trying to offer some hope. "And we could begin as soon as today if you want. Though it's understandable if you need to think about it, maybe talk it over with your precinct."

"How much will chemotherapy help?"

"That's the problem—it may not help at all. We have drugs that work against this type of cancer, we know doses and side effects, but there's no guarantee. And even if it does help, it may help slow the cancer only for a few months."

"I don't want the treatment to make her sick."

"Neither do I. Her quality of life is the most important thing. There's a small chance she could have some stomach upset, but fortunately, the majority of dogs don't experience ill effects from treatment. Chemotherapy for this disease can be given in a pill form or as an IV injection."

I review the various chemotherapy protocols, the schedule of administration, and the costs. Franny, being a service dog, will receive a discount if Officer Nelson elects chemotherapy. I give him a handout with more detail on everything we've just discussed—hearing about these options for the first time can be a lot to take in, and the handout will make it easier for Officer Nelson to share the information with his police chief and with his family.

At the end of my spiel he asks, "Will she still be able to smell? I've heard that people's sense of smell can be altered. She's a working dog, and she needs to be able to smell just as good as now. My captain won't pay for her out of the budget if she can't do search and rescue."

"I don't know," I begin, trying to be completely transparent. "I'm sorry, but we don't have a readily available way to measure just how much a dog on chemotherapy can smell and if those scents are altered in any way. But I can tell you I've never had a pet parent complain that their dog has had any issue with smell. And I've treated other police dogs that never seemed to miss a beat when back on the job."

I wait while he weighs this information.

"So how will we know?" he asks, seemingly just thinking out loud. "I guess we'll just have to see how she does." His voice trails off.

Officer Nelson shakes my hand and thanks me for my time. He plans to take Franny back to police headquarters to present this data to his chief, and then to discuss the situation with his wife. He promises to call me with his decision.

Three days after I first met Franny, I hear over the loud-speaker, "Line five, Mr. Nelson with Franny. Line five."

I pick up the receiver and say, "Hello. How's Franny?"

"She's doing fine, thanks," Officer Nelson begins. "But I have some more questions."

"Okay. Please go ahead."

"So, I've been reading over the handout. Which of these protocols do you think's best?"

"Again, there's not *one* that's better than another. It just depends on whether you want to give her a pill each day and bring her in here to recheck once a month, or if you want her to come in once a week for many weeks for an IV injection. The chance of the chemotherapy working is unknown. Her cancer could respond to none of the protocols, to all of them, or only to some. But it's impossible to know until we try. Trial and error, really. I know the uncertainty can be really hard, but there's no wrong answer here. The goal of treatment is to attempt to slow her mast cell tumor while giving her good quality months."

"But which do you think is best?"

"There isn't one that's better. There's no wrong option here. On some level, the pills would be the easiest for her, because she won't have to come in as often. And if they don't work, we could always try the injections."

There's silence on the other end of the phone.

"Okay, thanks. I'll think about it," Officer Nelson says. And then he hangs up.

The next day I receive another call from the policeman.

"Did you decide what you want to do?" I ask.

"I have a couple more questions. Which protocol do you think's best for Franny? And how will we know if it's working?"

I sit down and take a deep breath, knowing how difficult this discussion is for any dog parent.

"We can't really know which will be best," I begin. "They might all work or, unfortunately, none of them could do much, remember? The only way we'll know it's working is if the mass doesn't come back for a while. When the mass grows back, it means it is no longer working. And the most important thing to remember is that we can't cure this type of cancer."

I don't want to be so blunt, but clearly, I'm having trouble getting through.

"What about her nose? My chief says she has to be able to work, and for that she has to be able to smell."

"I realize that. But that's another unknown. Her sense of smell could be altered, but dogs have three hundred million olfactory receptors in their noses compared to our six million. So even if she loses some, there's still a chance she'd be able to track just fine. The other police dogs I've treated have been okay. But again, nothing's for certain."

"Yeah, but this is tracking in a field, sometimes through marshes, and into woods. It's not easy work. And it is physically strenuous. Will she be able to keep up?"

"Most dogs are able to go about their daily activities with no issues. I have some dogs on chemo that still compete in agility or in obedience trials. I've had other dogs that work for the Seeing Eye who are still able to lead their owners."

"Thanks. I'll tell the chief. But I still don't know what we're going to do."

Officer Nelson hangs up, and I reach for my stack of charts, getting ready to see my afternoon appointments before the weekend.

"Hey, Doc," Tiara asks as she walks toward the oncology treatment area. "Um, we, ah, have a family who just walked right in with their dog wanting to see you. But they don't have an appointment."

"Just offer them an appointment, please. Whenever my next available opening is. And then please get their records from their regular vet."

"I did. I mean, I tried. When I told the family that you don't have any availability until next week, they burst out crying." A tortured look is on her face.

"Hmm," I breathe out, mulling over the situation. "If you can get the records ASAP, and if the family doesn't mind waiting, I can try to fit them in."

With that, Tiara heads back up front. Ten minutes later, she presents me with records for Lucky Stewart, a seven-year-old mixed-breed dog. Lucky has had a full workup to include blood work, chest X-rays, an abdominal ultrasound, and a biopsy from a mass in his hindquarters. After reviewing all of these, I call up to the front desk, asking Tiara to walk the family into my exam room.

With a light tap on the door, I enter the exam room to be greeted by a family of five plus their dog. I am a little taken aback. I was not expecting such a large group! There is barely enough room left for me. I feel their collective stare.

Lucky is perched on his pet parent's lap, a shaggy beige midsized dog, panting. He reminds me of Benji, from the movies.

"Thank you so much for waiting, I'm Doctor—"

"You've got to save him!" Mrs. Stewart interrupts. "He means everything to us!" Her husband puts a hand on her shoulder. "He truly means everything to us," she repeats, a little more calmly this time.

I smile warmly. "Yes, our four-legged members are a very important part of our family. I understand. What I'd like to do first is—" Again, I'm interrupted.

"No, Doc, you don't understand. Lucky has saved our lives."

I look around and all eyes are still on me. Each family member is nodding, as if to the beat of music I cannot hear. I pause, waiting to see if there are more details to follow.

Mrs. Stewart's hand is shaking as she rummages through her purse. She pulls out a crumpled newspaper article. She offers it to me, her hand still shaking. I am a bit leery to take it, as there is a butterscotch candy stuck to the paper. But I do not want to be rude. Seriously, where are latex gloves when you need them? I look down at the paper.

Dog Saves Family's Life in Tragic Fire

Looking back at the family of five, I see tears streaming down all their faces. Mr. Stewart's shoulders are heaving as he silently cries. Mrs. Stewart remains a bit more composed.

"He saved us. We were all asleep in bed. We didn't know that the house was burning. I, I don't even know why we didn't hear the smoke detectors." The woman looks down at the floor, then glances up at me with blue eyes filled with sadness. "And he woke us up. Lucky woke us up." With that, she wipes the tears from her eyes and blows her nose. I hand her another tissue. "So, you see, he saved us. Now we need to save him." The woman pets her dog's head.

I take a step back. I get it now. After I explain about their dog's cancer, anal gland carcinoma, and treatment options, the family, in jumbled unison, elect treatment. But given that Lucky recently had surgery, he will need to wait another week to fully heal. I assure the Stewart clan that it is in Lucky's best interest to heal first and then begin treatment. The family exits my exam room, a bit lighter as they go.

I arrive at the office Monday morning and see a handwritten phone message taped to my computer screen: "Officer Nelson wants to ask more questions."

It's 7:00 a.m., too early to call him back, which is good. I'll need to be fully awake to answer the same questions yet again.

I go through my morning appointments without issue. When I come back to my computer, I find that I have a stack of phone messages. It's lunchtime, so I sit down to return all these calls. I speak with a woman who asks me about cloning her cat (I don't do that), and then with a gentleman who asks about some "medicine" he found on the internet. Then I dial Officer Nelson's number.

"Hello. Sorry I missed your call," I begin. "You said you have more questions?"

"We've decided to treat," he announces. "I think we're going to go the intravenous route, if that's okay?"

"Sure. That's great that you decided. I can pass you along to the receptionist to make an appointment."

"Can we start today? It's been weeks since she had the surgery. I don't want to give it any more time to grow back."

"Sure, we'll find some time to fit her in," I say. Then I transfer the call to the front desk staff. Because my service is fully booked, the best Tiara can do is something at the tail end of the day. (That's a little veterinary humor: tail end of the day.)

At 5:00 p.m., Officer Nelson arrives with Franny, her nose gliding over the ground, sniffing all the way, and leaving a trail of drool behind her, outlining the path she's taken. The man in blue is obviously nervous for his partner as he hands the oncology technician the dog's leash. Franny lags behind her, taking in new scents along the way to the treatment room in back.

I reach for the canister where the biscuits are kept, and Franny jumps to attention. *That* she smells easily. A bubble begins to form from her long right jowl, and then a few drops of saliva hit the floor. Please don't shake your head, girl, or all of that drool will go flying. I quickly give her a treat so that she doesn't have time to shake.

Cassidy walks the dog up onto the scale: seventy-four pounds. Franny is thin for her breed, but that's because of the cancer. Ideally, she'll respond favorably to the chemotherapy and put on a few pounds.

After I calculate her dose, Jackie prepares the drugs. The two other oncology nurses lay Franny on her side, telling her that she's a good girl. The bloodhound needs to hold still only for about fifty seconds, but we can see that she likes the attention and would happily lie on the treatment table much longer. The tech chooses a vein on Franny's left hind leg. She daubs alcohol on the dog's short reddish fur, then inserts the butterfly catheter. Franny doesn't move. She has large veins that are easy to stick, and the technician can then inject the chemotherapy into the catheter, which carries it into the vein.

Once we're done, Franny stands up and gives a full-body shake, which sends the drool flying. Cassidy makes pretend gagging sounds as she reaches for the paper towels. With no remorse, Franny trots out with Jackie to Officer Nelson, who seems delighted to have his partner back by his side.

The K-9 team returns seven days later. As long as everything goes well, we'll be seeing Franny and her partner once a week for four treatments, then once every two weeks for four treatments, then once every three weeks thereafter. Officer Nelson smiles as he enters the waiting room and checks in at the front desk.

"How did Franny do this week?" I ask.

"She did well," he answers, once again wiping Franny's face. "You couldn't even tell she'd had chemo. I was hesitant to work her at first, but she did just fine."

This is good news. I begin to lead Franny back to the treatment area, but then she leads me around the corner, heading straight for the canister of biscuits. Yep—her nose and her memory are working just fine. And she's tall enough to rest her head on the counter as she looks longingly at the container.

"Franny, come here," the tech says, coaxing the dog onto the scale. Franny leaves a small puddle of drool on the counter where her head has been. After her weigh-in, she sits still to have her blood drawn. The tech gives her a few biscuits for being such a good patient, which only causes her to drool more. While the blood sample is being analyzed, I perform a physical. Everything looks good, and Franny's gained two pounds. No surprise with the way she seems to inhale the goodies. After receiving her second treatment, the bloodhound ambles out to the waiting room with the technician. Reunited, the police team leaves to head back to the precinct.

At Franny's fourth treatment, Officer Nelson tells us that whenever he and Franny are coming to the clinic, as soon as they get within a couple of turns of our parking lot, Franny beings to whine excitedly in the back of the squadron SUV. It's as if she has her own internal GPS.

Today is no different from her previous appointments—
the canine pulls Cassidy to the back, heading straight for the
biscuits. For this visit, though, we have an abdominal ultrasound scheduled in order to get a good view of her stomach,
and to make sure that the tumor isn't growing back. It takes
three people to lift the dog up onto the table. Girlfriend has
put on some weight—she's now up to ninety-four pounds,
twenty more than when she started chemotherapy. The internist puts the gel and cold probe onto the dog's abdomen and
spends several minutes looking and searching, but comes up
with nothing. Thankfully, Franny has no evidence of any cancer regrowth. We lift Franny off the table, and then she and
I, along with my tech team, head back to the oncology area
to begin her blood work, physical exam, and chemotherapy
treatment. And biscuits! Franny never lets us forget to give
her biscuits.

I head out to the waiting room to tell Officer Nelson the
good news.

"Guess who's gained more weight? But don't say me!" I
add with a wink. I think I'd seriously burst into tears if he'd
guessed me.

"Oh, no, how much does she weigh?"

"She's gained twenty pounds since we first started treatment! Looks like she's making up for lost time. But the best
news is that her ultrasound is completely normal. There's no
sign of her cancer."

He's smiling ear to ear, and now his cheeks become flush, and his eyes get a little misty.

"After today, we can space out Franny's treatments to every other week," I add.

I take the afternoon off from work to head into the city for a series of my own medical tests. They're all routine, but with a serious purpose—to make sure there's still no evidence of the *C* word for me.

Mike picks me up from work and drives me in. I don't make it easy for him, but he insists. Which is to say, I'm not exactly panting with eager anticipation like Franny. In fact, I'm very nervous—okay, cranky—whenever I have a battery of tests like this. But does anyone look forward to being poked and prodded?

My veins don't bulge like Franny's, so I worry they won't be able to easily hit one. Then I worry that, even if they access my vein, another clot will form from the IV catheter for the contrast dye for the CT scans.

Mostly, though, I worry about the results, with what-ifs again swirling in my head. Franny has the great advantage of her species, which is living fully in the moment. No regrets, no what-ifs. Officer Nelson knows what worry is all about, but his dog does not. Worrying never changes an outcome; it simply wears out the worrier. Or warrior in this case.

It gives me some comfort to know that the staff of the cancer treatment center are at the top of their game, and that they'll be able to give me all my test results today, before I go home. So at least my what-ifs won't hang over me all week. Even so, the tests take hours. After my blood work, the nurse gives me contrast dye to drink—a viscous liquid they offer in a variety of flavors, all designed to try to disguise the fact that the stuff tastes terrible. I'm given an hour to gag it all down, but type A that I am, I drink it in fifteen minutes. I'm given intravenous contrast dye as well, but at least that doesn't involve my taste buds.

After all this prep, I undergo three CAT scans. Then I get back into my street clothes and meet with two different doctors on my team. It is a long day, but thank all the heavens in all of the worlds, the news is good. Actually, it's great. There is no evidence of that *C* word.

I drift out of the clinic on a cloud of gratitude, relief, and optimism. For the first time in months, I can allow myself to think about seeing my son grow up and get married, maybe my becoming a grandma, having "golden years" to spend with Mike. But just to show that God has a wicked sense of humor . . .

On our way out of the cancer center, Mike is slightly ahead of me, walking at a brisk pace as we approach the hospital parking garage. With Kansas a distant memory, he's no longer timid about crossing streets in Manhattan. Exhausted from the day's big events, I'm lagging behind, but my husband is eager to pay the parking fee before there's a line, get back to our car, then maybe escape Manhattan before the worst of the rush-hour traffic sets in.

Compared to yesterday, I now feel that I have all the time in the world; I don't see why we should hurry—we're sure to be sitting in hideous traffic whether we leave now or an hour from now.

In a feeble attempt to catch up to Mike, I step off the curb, then maybe walk three steps when all of a sudden—BAM! I stumble back a few steps, dropping my purse. One of the parking attendants has backed right into me! I'm stunned but, luckily, not seriously hurt. But boy, am I mad! With steam coming out of my ears—it's as if he'd smashed into my radiator—I pick up my handbag and give the car a good whack with it. Damned if I'll survive surgery, radiation therapy, chemotherapy, and the C word, only to be taken out by this doofus who never looked where he was going. I make him roll down the passenger side window so that I can tell him exactly what I think of his driving abilities in a loud, take-no-prisoners voice. Mike watches in horror, then ducks into the parking garage as if to say, "Who, me? I'm not with that crazy lady."

The driver admits that he hadn't looked before going in reverse. I assure him that, if he'd killed me, I would have (insert choice swear word here) haunted him for all eternity. His eyes get very big, and I suspect he's praying as we speak.

Eventually, I move on, then get into our car, safe and sound.

Getting hit happened so quickly—it was something I never anticipated and never could have controlled. But it was a valuable lesson. You worry yourself sick over testing and the C word, then get run over on the way home. Fact is, if you're living in the moment, not regretting the past or worrying about the future, you might still have a serious illness, but you're less likely to let a bad driver back into you.

Before the C word, I'd always thought that life was so under my control, and yet the disease has helped me realize that I was never in control of the really big things, or even the medium things. I close my eyes as a tear rushes down my cheek, grateful my tests were good, thankful to be alive, thankful not to be in the hospital with a broken leg, like the gray/white cat Sultan, back at the clinic. Before too long, I nod off to sleep.

Two weeks go by, and I'm still feeling good thanks to my clean bill of health. I've also mentally recovered from my "near-death" experience in the parking lot.

Officer Nelson brings Franny in for her next chemotherapy treatment. As the dog rounds the corner to our oncology treatment area, I notice that her body has definitely filled out, maybe a bit too much, since we started her protocol. The dog steps up onto the scale. She weighs exactly one hundred pounds! My team puts on the Commodores' "She's a Brick House" and turns the volume up. After doing her blood work, physical exam, and intravenous injection, I take her back to the waiting room to brief Officer Nelson.

"I can't believe she's gained more weight," he says, taking the canine's leash. "But down at the station everyone's been giving her treats."

"That's okay. It's better than the opposite, right? We have a dog with terminal cancer who's on chemotherapy and has gained twenty-six pounds, but who's counting? It's a good sign."

He looks down lovingly at his canine companion. Then he says, "Nearly forgot. Did you see the news? I brought this for you." He hands me an article clipped from the newspaper.

Police Dog Helps Lead Investigators Toward Hit-Run Killer

A police dog helped authorities identify the hit-and-run driver who killed a woman waiting for a bus. Police in the county specifically reached out for Franny because of the bloodhound's extreme tracking skills. Law enforcement credited Franny with picking up their investigation and leading them toward the suspect. Franny was able to track the driver from the crime scene to where he used further transportation to flee, the chief said . . .

I reach down to pet the dog. "Way to go, Franny! You're such a good girl. You're a hero!" I'm delighted that the chemo has not interfered with the bloodhound's crime-stopping career. If that guy in the parking lot had really flattened me, then taken off, maybe Franny would have been the one to track him down.

Every year our state holds an Animal of the Year Award Assembly. Anyone can fill out the application and write an essay as to why they think a certain pet is worthy of this honor. Categories are based on the type of animal: dog, cat, horse, pocket pet—whatever.

Many months have gone by, and Franny has beaten the odds with her cancer, and I feel that, because of her continued work in the community, she would be a good candidate for the award. But first, I need to ask permission from her police partner. When Officer Nelson arrives for Franny's appointment, I tell him. He says that he's honored on her behalf and very grateful on his own.

It's eight months since we started treating this canine, and she's due for a repeat ultrasound before today's chemo. With bated breath, I wait for the results. Even if Franny has recurrent disease, I would still nominate her, though it would be bittersweet. My team comes back from internal medicine with Franny trailing behind, her nose, as always, hovering just off the ground. I read the ultrasound report: another good evaluation. The police dog receives her treatment and a few more biscuits. Then she's off for more search-and-rescue missions until her next appointment.

"Hey, Doc, did you see this?" Cassidy hands me her cell phone. Though we haven't seen Franny in two weeks, the tech follows the police dog's Facebook page. A child had wandered off, and after family, friends, and the local police failed to find her, Franny and Officer Nelson were called in to save the day. Franny's a hero yet again!

"That is awesome!" I say beaming. "I should call him." With that, I dial his number.

"Hey, Doc, how's it going?" says the police officer, recognizing our hospital number on his phone.

"Oh, I'm calling to congratulate you and Franny for finding that little girl. That dog is amazing!"

"Yeah, she did great. What they didn't mention was how she tracked that scent for hours. It was exhausting, and we both got cut up in the woods, but Franny stayed right on it."

I could hear the pride in his voice. He and Franny are partners in every sense of the word, and together they accomplish far more than either could accomplish alone.

"Oh, and did you hear?" he adds, almost as an afterthought. "Franny won Dog of the Year!"

"That's amazing! No one told me. I would have thought they'd tell the person who nominated her. But I'm so glad she won! She absolutely deserves it."

"They want to do a photo shoot. And a video," Officer Nelson tells me. "With you, at the hospital."

I'm not one for being in front of the camera, but this is for a good cause, one that will show people how well a dog can do on chemotherapy. "Sure, I'm happy to help. Just let me know the dates."

It turns out that the awards committee wants to have the video play during the assembly when each recipient receives their honor. A cameraman and an interviewer show up at my office the following day—so much for plenty of notice. They interview me, video Franny, and take photographs of my oncology crew along with the officer and his canine partner. Evidently, Franny likes the limelight. Officer Nelson diligently wipes away her drool. The film crew and the police team then leave to drive to a field to video Franny in action, finding Officer Nelson's "lost" wife, Alice, who's very pregnant. Fortunately, her plight is merely staged for the camera, but it makes for a fun video that demonstrates Franny's amazing nose.

Officer Nelson continues to bring Franny in every few weeks for her chemotherapy. The hero-dog now weighs 105 pounds, but the weight doesn't appear to concern her in the least. Not so for me. I've gained twenty pounds since beginning my treatment, which I'm told is "chemo weight." I get upset if I gain a few pounds normally, so this side effect is not something I'm able to take in stride. Moreover, I didn't eat my way to this number on the scale—at least there might have been some pleasure in that. Maybe it's just the universe having a good laugh. No matter how much food I resist or how many miles I walk, these pounds remain very loyal—they don't want to go anywhere without me.

On the anniversary of Franny's first appointment, I sit down next to Officer Nelson in the exam room to have a happy, though serious, chat.

"We've been treating Franny for a full year now," I start out. "And she's done incredibly well. Certainly, she's beaten the odds."

"Yes. And we have you to thank for that."

"Well, I'm delighted that she's done so well. But I bring up where we are timewise because some people would stop treatment at this point. We could continue, though we can't say that further chemo would be of any benefit."

"Won't the cancer just come right back?"

"We're in unchartered territory right now—which is a good thing, because it means she's done much better than expected. But we've always known it will come back. The question is how soon. Her initial prognosis was only a few months, and now we're at a year."

I pause for a moment, knowing that I'm getting into very delicate territory.

"The negatives of continued treatments are the time it takes to come in, the expense to your police department, and, most of all, the risk that it could wear out her bone marrow."

Officer Nelson looks at me as if he's not quite sure he understands.

"The marrow is where she makes her red blood cells, white blood cells, and platelets. We always do blood work to make sure these are fine, that we're being safe. But eventually, the drugs can put too much strain on her bone marrow and lower her cell counts. It may not happen, but if it does, it could be very serious."

The officer sits and thinks for a moment. "It's not about the money. And you've been so kind to give us a discount on everything. It really helps, and my chief appreciates it."

"Well, she does so much to help the public. Just like you. We're very grateful to you both."

Glancing away, blushing slightly, the officer says, "Well, it's no problem to come in for the treatments. Franny loves those treats—she gets so excited whenever the SUV gets near the hospital. Plus, she's not had any issues with her blood work, right?"

I nod, waiting for his decision.

"Let's go ahead. I realize we can't know if it's going to help, but I want to do whatever I can for my partner."

Franny and Officer Nelson continue to come in once every month for chemotherapy. Periodically, we repeat an abdominal ultrasound to make sure her cancer is still in a remission and, thankfully, it is.

"Hey, Doc," the policeman says, seeing me across the waiting room.

I walk over to say hello.

"I have some good news," he continues. "Alice had the baby! It's a boy!"

"That's wonderful," I say, and give him a congratulatory hug. Then the proud father shows me pictures of their new addition. I ooh and ah, then say, "Please tell your wife that I say congratulations."

"I have more news," he adds. "Franny is officially retired!"

"What?! Why?" I'm baffled. "Did something happen? I thought she loved to work?"

"She does. It's just that it's been too much for her lately. She's gained so much weight that it's hard to run for hours. Navigate the woods . . . jump through marshes. But it's all good. She's happy—fat and happy! The best part is that she gets to live with us and our new baby."

He rubs the dog's face. Franny now tips the scales at 119 pounds, which makes her lumber and jiggle when she walks. It's hard to imagine her continuing on as an action-adventure star, but now she'll have a wonderful retirement in a very loving home. And certainly, the Nelsons won't ever have to worry that their young son will get lost.

I hear from the Nelsons periodically, and I'm delighted that Franny continues to do well in civilian life. She's never lost any of the weight she gained during her chemotherapy treatment, though it doesn't seem to bother her. The bottom line is that she's happy. She could be a lesson for all of us—especially me.

Since developing my weight gain, I struggle with being happy, even though my medical team tells me that it has nothing to do with overindulgence. It's a late-term side effect from my treatment called lymphedema, which is swelling in a part of one's body due to accumulated fluid, specifically lymphatic fluid. It can happen if lymph nodes are removed, or if a person receives a fair amount of radiation, or from surgery. I've had all three, so it's not really surprising that I'd add a few pounds. The diagnosis should let me off the hook for guilty feelings; on the other hand, it means that no amount of exercise and disciplined eating is going to help.

The lymphedema in my arms from the blood clots and the vasculitis initially seems to have gotten a little better, but now we seem to be at some sort of standstill. Worse, I have lymphedema on my abdomen/pelvis and thighs, so much so that I've needed to buy a new wardrobe. I try not to look in the mirror because, right now, my body makes me profoundly sad. The swelling also plays into my short suit of patience. I'm told it can take a long time to improve, but nothing good will happen if I don't try. I plan to work with a lymphedema specialist, approaching fluid reduction with renewed vigor and all the ingenuity I can muster. But for that, I have to stay positive.

Luckily, when I'm working at the clinic, I don't have time to feel bad for myself. And when I'm helping my animal patients, they never notice how I look. I feel whole—perfectly okay as is—whenever I'm with them, and on top of that, they thank me for my help with a wag of a tail or a sloppy, wet kiss. They don't see my worth as being inversely proportional to the circumference of my thighs, or the size of my dress. This is one of the many lessons I'm trying to learn from my furry patients.

9

NEWTON, PART THREE

My friend Jim died two days ago. He was my age, and he got his diagnosis about five months before I got mine. He never had surgery or radiation, just an awful lot of chemotherapy, and through it all, he kept working. He said he did it for his family, to try to leave them as well off as he could, even though it took a big toll on him. Jim did experience a peripheral neuropathy, where his hands and feet remained in a numb sensation. I know it made it difficult for him to do his job as a top-notch tennis coach. I hadn't seen Jim since I began treatment, but I wanted to, and I offered to come by, but by that point he didn't want to be seen. The *C* word was wearing out his body. We did manage some very meaningful phone conversations, though, for which I am very grateful. It's always good to commiserate with someone who understands, who's walked in your shoes, or in this case, your slippers.

Newton is much quieter in the house these days. If it weren't for my son practicing piano in the background, you could hear a pin drop. Newton used to get excited when Peter played the piano. He'd get out one of his Nylabones and chew on it or begin to play with a plush toy—though his idea of playing with a toy was more like eviscerating it. But not today. No longer do we have white cotton fluff all over the carpet from Newton's latest conquest. Today, Newton watches as I do some light housework, but my dog doesn't follow me around anymore—he trails me only with his eyes. He prefers to spend his days lying in one of his five dog beds that have been placed strategically around the house. Thankfully, he is not in any pain; he just doesn't feel like doing anything. Which is another way of saying that he's not having a very meaningful quality of life.

Peter stops playing piano, realizing his "big brother" is missing from the action. He goes to Newtie in his dog bed and lies with him, stroking his head. Newton gives Peter's face one gentle lick. The boy wipes the wetness off of his cheek with the back of his hand. Though it's time for Newton's dinner, I don't want to do anything to break up this tender moment. I wait for my son to get up from the floor before picking up Newtie's bowl.

Lately, Newton's regular dog food is not so enticing to him.

I reach for the bag instinctively but then I put the scooper back, mostly full. Newton prefers to have canned dog food mixed in with the kibble, but I am now also adding some lunch meat, hoping to coax my dog to eat a little more. The turkey cold cuts have been working well enough, but today I decide to cook something special. I may not be able to control how much Newton eats, and I certainly can't control the disease process, but I sure as heck can make delicious food for my boy to enjoy during these last days. I roast an entire chicken, then brown a pound and a half of hamburger meat, being careful to drain off any of the oils lest I give him diarrhea. I then make a large pot of white rice to add to the proteins. I don't have to worry about counting carbs; I just want my boy to eat. I take the chicken off the bone and put it in Tupperware alongside the Tupperware filled with ground burger and rice.

Then I call my husband on his cell.

"Hi. What's up?" I can tell he's busy at work.

"Can you bring home dinner tonight?"

"Sure, but what happened to the chicken? I thought you were going to make chicken?"

"I did. But that's for the dog." I pause, waiting for a remark that does not come. "And so is the hamburger. And so is the rice. They're all in the refrigerator and they're all for him." I have carefully labeled each plastic container with a big FOR NEWTON! DO NOT EAT! in black Sharpie marker. I hear a sigh, but I know that Mike understands how much pleasure this gives me.

Our boxer, Newton, is the dearest of friends, and an integral part of our family, but the *C* word is taking a toll on his body. I know we'll soon be faced with a terrible decision that I've helped so many families face. The hardest part is the timing, which all comes down to the animal's quality of life. Is he still eating? Does she want to be with you? Is she in any pain? No one wants to make that dreadful decision even one day too late, because no one wants their four-legged family member to suffer. But we don't want to lose a beloved pet one day earlier than we have to, either. It's different in human medicine. The day a human loved one is to end their time here is not our decision, at least not in this country, not at this time.

My motto for battling the *C* word is that I never give up, and I certainly never give in. Yes, feel sorry for my husband when he and I bicker, because I won't necessarily back down, especially if I am convinced that I am right. But in Newton's case, for our family, the humane thing is to realistically assess when the battle has been lost and to let him go. We're doing palliative care for our dog now, which is care meant to help a patient have an improved quality of time without increased quantity of time. For Newtie, this means that we give him prednisone, a steroid pill, to try to help with the swelling of his lymph nodes. It means he gets to eat people food when he was only ever allowed dog food. And it means he can come up and cuddle with us on some of the furniture when he was always relegated to his own dog bed or the carpeted floor.

Somehow, it no longer bothers me that his slobber might get on the upholstery.

Three days go by. We continue our usual routine. Newton rests comfortably in his dog bed in our bedroom. My son is downstairs practicing for a piano concert—Mozart and Chopin, the light stuff. Mike is packing a small suitcase for a business trip, which will keep him out of town for a couple of nights. The work trip, though it will have him busy with a study for a new ocular medication, does give Mike a reprieve from the gloom in our household. With everything going on here, however, I'm worried about him being gone.

"I hate to leave with Newton this way," he tells me.

"I know. Let's just hope he'll be okay." I go over to Newton in his dog bed to give him some love. Then, over my shoulder, I say, "I know you have to go. It's not like you can get out of it."

"Trust me, I tried. But I feel terrible leaving you with this . . . with him like this. Do you think he'll be okay until I get back?" He fiddles nervously with the zipper on his bag.

"I hope so. Maybe he will. He's been stable the last few days." It's a strange thing. The other times when we were faced with a decision about euthanizing a pet, Mike wasn't around. He was there to help in the decision process—we both only want the best for our beloved animals. But it was too much for Mike to bear to be physically present at the sad time at the end of life. Some people can't be present. And that is okay. It is a personal choice, with no wrong answer.

Mike and I are silent for a moment. Neither of us wants to talk about what we need to talk about.

"But if he takes a turn, are you okay if we need to make a decision and you aren't here?"

There. I've put it on the table. But my question is met with silence. Mike sits down on the edge of the bed, and I sit down next to him. It's a very somber moment. I reach for my husband's hand.

After a moment, he says, "Yeah. I mean, how could you not go ahead if things get worse. I don't want Newtie to suffer. I'd feel so bad for him. But I should be with you and Peter. I don't want you to have to go through that alone."

Mike looks at me, the tears welling up in his eyes. We embrace for a long time, seated on the bed.

Days go by. Newton has been sleeping in our bed with me all night. That third morning, I feel his warm breath as he yawns. He raises his head and looks around, as if he can't believe that morning has come so soon. This dog definitely likes the comforts of human bedsheets and blankets. He's curled up on Mike's pillow, slobber and all. Nothing a load of wash can't fix. We head downstairs to begin our day.

It's summer now, and school is just out. Mornings are a little slower, much less frenetic. My son comes downstairs in his pajamas, yawning as he enters the kitchen.

"Hi, Newtie Putie," he says, patting his dog's head. I throw him a smile.

"Hungry? Want something to eat?"

"I thought all the food in the fridge was for the dog?" he says, giving me a devilish smile.

"Ha, ha, not funny. Newtie has his groceries, we have ours. You want something or not?"

"I'm good," and with that, my two-legged boy heads to the basement for some serious time with his Xbox. Newton stays with me in the kitchen, nestled in his dog bed.

When I reach down for his dog bowl, our boxer doesn't seem to notice. Evidently, this morning I'll have to pull out all the stops to make his breakfast irresistible. Lately, he's preferred ground beef to poultry, so I put some burger in his bowl with some of the rice. For kicks, I add a bit of gravy from last night's dinner, then pop the whole ensemble into the microwave. Warmer, smellier food is always more enticing than cold food for a pet, especially one that has a poor appetite. It doesn't smell half bad, I must admit. I set the bowl down in its usual spot. Newton raises his head, then settles back down. Sigh.

In a sweet, coaxing tone I say, "Newtie, come here, honey. Want your breakfast?" The dog doesn't move. I bring the food bowl over to him and set it down.

"Newtie, breakfast," I say again. He looks at me as if he understands what I want him to do. He stands up, arches his back in a stretch, then gingerly eats a few bites. I swear he is eating just to please me, just to be my good boy. It works; I love him for trying. After a few nibbles, he's done. I wipe his face and he lies back down.

It's never easy to say goodbye to a loved one. Through good days and bad, our pets provide such unconditional love, support, and companionship. They're with us for fun times, and also are there to snuggle with when the outside world seems too harsh. Newton has been all of these things to all three of us in our family. But just as he has made our lives better, we must make his life as good as we can, right to the last moment. I remind myself of what I review with other pet parents when they are nearing the end of life with their cat or dog.

- *Is my pet in pain?* Veterinary prescription pain medication can help.
- *Is my pet eating?* Offering other tasty foods or an appetite stimulant may help. Subcutaneous fluids may help with hydration if needed.
- *Is my pet active?* Lethargy and sleeping a lot more than usual are signs that the disease is taking its toll.

- *Is my pet comfortable?* Does he/she have the soft bedding that they like; is the room temperature appropriate? Sometimes veterinary prescribed anti-inflammatory medications can help.
- *Is my pet happy?* Does he/she still want to be with me or does he/she go off alone? This is also another sign that the disease is progressing.

I try to block out my thoughts. If only for a bit. I sweep the kitchen floor and put a couple of stray glasses into the dishwasher. I go upstairs to wash the sheets, then put a clean set on the bed. But I've stalled long enough. I need to do a physical exam on my beloved dog. I head downstairs to find Newtie right where I left him, lying in his dog bed, asleep.

I gently wake Newton and get him to stand up. Then I give him a rubdown, which I can tell feels good to him. I go deep into his neck, then segue into my physical examination as he holds still like a good boy. I feel the lymph nodes under his neck, the ones in his shoulders, the ones in his axillary region, the ones in his groin, and the lymph nodes in the backs of his hind legs. They are all really big. Upon palpating his abdomen, I notice that his liver and spleen have enlarged as well.

"Peeeter!" I shout from the kitchen, down the basement stairs.

"Yeah?" my son shouts back.

"Can you come up here, please?" He must hear it in my voice.

Normally, I'd get an "Aw, Mom," or an "In a minute," which would last until I asked him again. And then maybe even a third reminder. But this time, Peter comes right up the stairs. He puts his arms around me, and we hug. We then sit on the floor next to our dog, my son petting his brindle brother.

"Honey," I begin, knowing this won't be an easy conversation. "Newtie's lymph nodes are really big. I'm worried about him. And even though I made him a delicious breakfast, he didn't want to eat it. And he has no energy at all."

Peter looks at me, his eyes searching my eyes, wishing there was another option. Finally, he says, "Mom, I know it's time."

How beautiful it is when our children surprise us with insight and wisdom, maturity and compassion, just when the universe calls.

"I know what we have to do." Then he adds, "I'm sorry, Newtie," as tears well up in his doe-like eyes.

"I'd have to take him into my work. Would you want to come?"

"Of course! I can't believe you even asked that."

"Okay. I just wanted to give you the option. Go get dressed and I'll call your dad." With that, Peter heads upstairs to get ready. I reach for the phone and dial Mike. I am dreading having to make this call. I hadn't expected Newton to take such a downward turn in only a few days. I had told Mike that I thought the dog would be okay while he was away. I was wrong.

I'm thankful that he picks up. When Mike's away on business, he doesn't always have the liberty of answering calls right when they come in.

"What's wrong? Is it Newton?" His voice is barely audible. "Give me a sec, let me step away from the group." I wait a moment, and hear a door shut. "What's going on?" he asks.

"Just what we were afraid of. It seems the minute you left, Newtie took a turn for the worse. I don't think he's enjoying his life, honey. He's just dragging through the hours. Barely eating. Barely moving."

I hear Mike breathing more heavily, perhaps even crying.

"O-okay," he gets out. Then we're silent for a moment.

I think about how to approach the topic gingerly, knowing that this will be hard on Mike from afar. But then I just say it.

"I think we need to euthanize him today. Waiting any longer is just making him suffer."

I hear Mike blow his nose.

"I know. Okay. I'm so sorry I can't be there for him. And for you and Peter. I should be there for both of you. Give Newtie a hug for me. And please tell Peter I love him." After a few moments, Mike adds, "Will you let me know when it's over?"

"Sure, I'll call you." Then, between tears, I whisper, "I love you."

"I love you, too."

I hang up the phone, blow my nose, then gather my things to go. I text my work team to alert them of our decision. The three of us head to the car, walking slowly. I scramble to find my phone in the bottom of my purse. I turn off its sound, for hearing an incessant series of dings, though likely my devoted work team replying, is too much to bear. I open the hatch to the back of my Audi wagon. Newton tries to jump in but is unsuccessful. I help raise up his back end and then slowly shut the door. I'd hope that Peter didn't see that, but he did. I've never seen him look so sad.

We do the twenty-minute drive to the hospital in complete silence, and it seems to take forever. Though the sun is out, we seem to be in a dense, gray fog. Finally, I pull into the parking lot, then go to the back to open the hatch for Newton. I put his leash around his neck, and then he hops out.

My son is still sitting in the car. Is he not going to come in after all? Have I missed a clue? As our dog and I go to the passenger side of the vehicle to check on him, Peter wipes his eyes and gets out. Then we trudge into the clinic together.

Tiara gives us a warm, knowing smile. No words are exchanged; they don't need to be. We've worked together for a long time and she understands, we speak in silence. As Newton, Peter, and I round the corner to the oncology section, Newton begins to slowly wag his little stump of a tail. This is a happy place for him. He grew up spending a lot of time here and knows the staff as friends. It is nice to see him happy. He has no fear; only friends are here.

"Newtie Patootie!" Cassidy says to the dog as she reaches down to pet him. Another technician, after realizing that we're in the building, comes down the hall to give me a hug. She wipes a tear from her eye. The internist sees us all and comes over. We don't have to tell him what's about to happen. He senses the sadness in the room, and he gives me a hug. The veterinary neurologist that I work with selflessly offers to be the one to give the injection. Politely, I decline. Though this is the hardest part of the job, it is my job to do all the same. I look to my son. I want him to feel the compassion that is surrounding us at this moment. Jackie gives Peter a quick embrace, then turns and looks at me. We both know that she cannot protect me from what we're facing. I give her a half-hearted smile and she puts her arms around me. We hug for a moment, but then I step back. I need to maintain some level of composure for the daunting task at hand.

"Peter, honey, let me know when you're ready," I say gently.

"It's okay, Mom. We can do it."

Hearing this, my coworkers begin to leave this space to give my son and me privacy. Jackie looks to me for direction—she knows this is not a one-person job. I stop the trio of oncology nurses and ask them to stay and help. They've been with my family every step of the way for Newtie's disease. And though it isn't easy for them, I know each one of them wants to be right there with us. Jackie hands me the necessary drugs and the IV catheter—my team began preparations as soon as I texted them. Just as I start to lower the table that Newton so often perched on top of, my dog tries to jump up on it, like he used to do. This time, though, he doesn't have the strength to make it, and he falls to the floor. I cringe. Peter goes to his rescue, putting a hand on his neck as the slightly stunned animal stands back up.

"Stay here, Newtie, wait. You're a good boy," he says. This is really difficult.

The table lowers and our dog steps on. As I raise the table back up, it is easy to see that he likes being up high. Silly boy. The technicians have Newton lie down. This position that he assumes is no different from the position he was in for all of the months during which he received chemotherapy. But there is no music playing in the background to accompany this moment.

"Are you okay, honey?" I ask my son, looking at him longingly. He nods a yes. Peter is stoic, standing at Newton's face, stroking the velvet-like wrinkles on the dog's forehead. I reach over and squeeze my brave son's hand.

Now the rest is on me. Euthanizing a pet, anyone's pet, is quite emotional. During this time with a family, I am so sad myself that I need to cry, yet I need to be present to comfort the grieving people as best I can. It's a very a difficult, heart-wrenching situation. I struggle to hold back my tears in order to see the vein in which I have to place a catheter. This time it's my own dog. And my son is here, whom I just want to hold and be a mom to. I'm walking a fine line, knowing that I must maintain composure to do a proper job, and yet I'm losing my own wonderful pet. I say a quick prayer, asking for the skill to put this catheter in with one try. No one can bear watching someone trying different veins to euthanize their animal. By the grace of God, the catheter goes in with the first stick. Forever trusting, Newtie does not move. He feels safe in this space.

He is set to receive two different medications. The first will be a tranquilizer overdose, so that he will go into a very deep sleep. The second injection will actually stop his heart and his lungs from working. The whole process may take only a minute or so. I look around the table. All four of the caring people around me have their eyes fixed on our dog. They do not see me looking at them. Tears flow down Cassidy's face. I take a deep breath and let the air out slowly. I can do this, I tell myself. Please, hands, keep steady, don't add any further worry to my son. I reach for the sedative, connect it to the catheter, and begin pushing it from the syringe into the vein. I softly talk to Newton as I am doing this: "Good boy, sweetheart," "Newtie is such a good boy," "We love you sooo much, good boy," I say. I look up to see Jackie with tears flooding down her face. I cannot look at any of the others or else I would lose it as well. Please, Lord, let me be able to do this. I look back down and take the next, the final, syringe. I hook this onto the catheter's opening and slowly begin giving my dog the drug. Moments seem forever. When the syringe is empty, I set it down and grab my stethoscope from around my neck to listen. He has no heartbeat; he has no breath. Newton has passed.

All three coworkers are crying. They step out of the room quickly, quietly, to give my son and me some time. He and I hug a deep, long hug. At first, he doesn't cry, but I know to hang on longer. Finally, with our continued embrace, he begins to weep, deeply, and of course I cry as well. It breaks my heart to see my son so brokenhearted. I don't let him go until his tears stop. My shoulder is wet with evidence of the love he has for his dog. We both turn to Newton's body lying on the table. Somehow one of my staff members has come in and covered him with a soft blanket. I never saw them do it, but I'm grateful for their kindness. Newton's head is not under the blanket. I tell my son I love him, and then we turn to pet our dog.

"I love you, too," he says. We stand in silence for a while. Then Peter gets a small twinkle in his eye.

"Remember when we first brought Newtie home as a puppy," he says, "and he peed right on my bedspread?"

I say, "And remember when he got so scared when that stranger who looked just like Uncle Fester from *The Addams Family* knocked on our door?"

"And remember how much he loved opening his birthday presents, shredding the tissue paper to find a squeaky toy?"

"And what about when he almost swallowed the squeaky! He loved those toys."

"And what about all those words you trained him to know,

214

Mom? I swear he was the only dog to know to back up when someone said 'excuse me.'"

"Yeah, he did have such a big vocabulary. He was such a good dog," I say, smiling.

"Yeah, he was."

"And he loved you so very much," I remind my son. "As hard as this was to do, we made the right decision. And you were so wonderful to be here with him. I know it wasn't easy. I'm very proud of you." We both hug again. "And I'm so very sorry. Do you want more time with Newtie right now?"

"No, I'm good. We can go."

Poking my head out of the door, I tell my staff that we'll be leaving. Crying unashamedly, each of them hugs each of us. I am grateful to work with such caring people, and I know they'll take care of Newton's body. It will take ten days to get his ashes back, but I'll deal with that when the time comes.

A great weight has been lifted off my shoulders. Though I am extremely sad, I was able to euthanize our dog with the dignity that he deserved. I was able, am able, to support my loving son, and he has handled a tough situation very well. As we walk through the waiting room to get to the parking lot, I feel all eyes heavy on us—the team of receptionists, dear Tiara's, and fellow pet parents, waiting for their names to be called. I'm in no shape to receive everyone's condolences, and I really just want to get back home with Peter. I keep my head down and we keep walking.

The drive home seems much faster, although Peter and I travel in silence once again. The sun casts a glare on the windshield as we pull into the driveway.

After we get out of the car and enter our home, the reality of the lonely void in our house sinks in. Funny how a single fifty-two-pound boxer can fill up a whole house. The happy reminiscing we did a half hour ago has quickly turned to such sorrow.

For a moment, we stand awkwardly in the kitchen, and then I share one more story. I tell Peter about the fawn boxer I had during vet school and residency, the one I was walking when I first met his father. Blitzen was incredibly special to me, my steadfast companion. I loved that dog so much that I used to beg him to live for many years, even though I knew the average life span for a boxer is nine years. I was fortunate; Blitzen lived until he was eleven. I was so sad after he passed, even though I knew that I had had two more years with my boy than the average boxer parent. Pets have a much shorter life span then we would ever choose for them. While I'd love to have had Blitzen for decades, I suppose the silver lining is that I got to experience a few or even many dogs in my lifetime.

"Each dog is different," I tell my son, "and each teaches us something different. And I think they are placed in our lives at different times, for just that purpose. It doesn't take away that this is hard and that it really hurts, but I promise you the pain will get better."

Peter looks at me, clearly understanding what I'm saying, but unable to say a word. We hug for just a moment. With that, my teenager heads to his room for some alone time, and I'm left by myself in the kitchen.

I often tell families that their pain and sorrow will get better. That it just takes time, and sometimes it takes a lot of time. I know it will get better for my family, for me, but right now those thoughts are not comforting. I am worn out and feel incredibly sad.

I reach for my phone to call Mike to tell him of the day's sad events.

10

DUSTY AND CALLIE

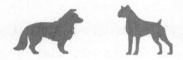

This visit to the cancer clinic marks the one-year anniversary of my battle against the *C* word. But this is not an anniversary anyone wants. Aren't such occasions supposed to involve dinner, candles, flowers? Mike is with me here today, but this situation is far from romantic. I have just completed blood work, three CT scans, a radiation oncologist appointment, and an audiologist appointment to check my ears, and I am tired. I take pride in being a good multitasker, but this is really exhausting.

Overall my stamina seems to have gotten better each month. I still have good days and not-so-good-days, but the degree of difference is thankfully less than in months past.

The more time that goes by with continued normal test results, the better.

Sitting impatiently in my medical oncologist's office, pending my results, I feel a flood of emotions, and I've never been a good swimmer. I've needed to cry a lot lately, but only a few tears leak out and then they stop. I am scared and nervous about getting past this milestone. Going in every three months for routine tests, it's as if I have to face my own mortality quarterly. And I am now waiting to see my medical oncologist. If the results are not what I'd like, I'll probably be in the gutter, or disappearing on a bender with cookies. Or potato salad. Or chip dip. But after I lick my wounds (and the spoon from the dip), I will remember that I'm a relentless warrior. Mike is next to me, my loyal comrade in arms. Today, I guess you could say he's my water wings. Either way, I'm very glad to have him by my side.

"Hey, Mike," I say, pulling him out of the trance that is his cell phone.

"Yeah?" He looks at me as he shifts his weight in the not-so-comfortable vinyl-covered waiting room chair.

"Have you had any thoughts about us getting a dog?" I ask him, though I'm not actually sure where I stand on the subject.

Since losing Newton, I have donated his dog food, toys, and all five dog beds to our local town shelter. At least they could go to helping a pet in need. Walking around our house, I still have very vivid memories of Newtie. I continue to look to places where he liked to lie, but, sadly, he's not there. At times I even find a few short, blunt hairs of his stuck in some fabric of the furniture. Despite my vigorous vacuuming, they are relentless. And I must admit, I have wrestled with feelings of guilt. Guilt that I'm here and my dog isn't. Guilt that maybe I could have done something different, something more, to help him to beat the *C* word. Guilt that in some crazy way, Newton gave it all up to save me.

"Funny you should mention it," my husband answers, pulling me out of my thoughts. "I've been thinking the same thing, just not sure yet that I'm ready."

We both sit in silence for a few minutes, contemplating this topic. In time there will be room in our hearts for a new dog, but first our hearts need to heal. None of this has been easy, and any decisions we make have to include Peter's desires as well. Even if our hearts aren't quite ready, if our son needs to give his love to another boxer, then we'll be there, ready to begin a new chapter together, as a family. But then the fears come rushing in. Will that new chapter include me? Will I still be around?

The receptionist comes to escort us to the exam room. I take a big gulp and squeeze my husband's hand.

We've had our share of scars recently, but we have come through them all a bit stronger and more loving for the wear. When the panic overtakes me, I ask myself this question: If I knew that everything was going to be okay, how would I act? Can I act that way now, even in the face of uncertainty? That would be taking a cue from my four-legged patients. They enjoy their time by living in the moment. They never waste their time, no matter how short or long, with worry.

I hear a soft knock on the exam room door, and it slowly opens. Mike grabs my hand, holding it tightly. My oncologist enters, standing tall in her starched white lab coat. I stare at her intently, trying to find some clue in her face as to whether she has good news or not such good news. She exchanges pleasantries with my husband, but I'm not listening to a word being said. Will her words of my results be my savior or my assassin? I want to shout, "Just tell me the results!"

She picks up on my anxiety and suddenly switches gears.

"Everything is fine," she says, looking at me with a broad smile. "Your tests are good."

Thank God. (Though I wish she could have skipped the pleasantries—and the suspense—and gone straight to the headline.) I dissolve into tears. Mike pats my knee. A pile of wet tissues accumulates on the chair next to me. I know big emotions make Mike uncomfortable, but this girl has to cry.

With tears in my eyes, I stand and ask if I can give my doctor a hug. She happily obliges, and we embrace, but for only a moment. I could have held on a lot longer, but it is not that sort of relationship. Mike stands up and strokes my back. In his comforting of me, I can feel him take a big sigh of relief. We all needed to hear good news. We all needed a reprieve from what life has dished out lately.

My doctor moves on to asking routine medical questions, which I struggle to answer while wiping my eyes and blowing my nose. The pile of wet tissues grows. At least I was given good news, really good news.

As the doctor talks, I ask myself again: How would I have acted if I'd known that everything would be okay? I would have been lighter and happier. I would have not taken myself or my situation so seriously. Now these answers are easy. But had I not worried so much about the results and trusted life's process a bit more, things could have been a lot more peaceful.

Maybe three months from now, when I face my next set of tests, I will approach them with this more placid outlook. Easier said than done, I know, but perhaps through baby steps, I can get there. I can practice when life throws me little speed bumps along the way: a leaky roof, my husband forgetting our real anniversary, my kid not turning in a homework assignment, a hard day at the office. If I'm being completely honest, despite my not being fully available to help (or nag, depending on your vantage point) during my treatment course, my son has managed to complete and submit his college applications. Our house didn't fall down. And Mike learned why we don't put a red shirt in with the white laundry.

As my husband and I gather our items to head home, I thank my doctor—she's given me back my life. Mike takes my hand as we leave the doctor's office. I give his hand a good squeeze in a show of appreciation for his support all along the way. He and I will go out for an early dinner tonight to cele-brate today's news—the way you do on a real anniversary.

I am so happy to be able to wholeheartedly return to work at my beloved clinic. Having been gone for a while certainly makes me appreciate the opportunity to be a veterinarian, and to work with such an amazing group of people. For me, it's more than a job—it's a big part of who I am. I'm back part-time, under my physician's recommendation, easing into it. Unfortunately, I get pretty tired toward the end of the day, and though I've tried to put boundaries up for myself with regard to the caseload, I need to follow through on these good intentions. Otherwise, I feel flat, like a cartoon character that got run over. I do not want to be Wile E. Coyote.

I walk into the clinic one ordinary morning, and Tiara greets me with a sly grin on her face, telling me there's something in ICU I'll want to check out. Even before going to my computer area to set down my belongings, I head to the back of the hos-pital, where I find four technicians bending over a large cage.

"Hey, Doc, you've gotta see this," an ICU tech says. The other three part to give me a better view.

"Oh, my goodness!" I let out. I kneel down and crawl into the cage, where a fawn-colored female boxer lies with a mess of puppies nuzzling her teats.

"When did she come in?" I ask.

"Last night. She was having trouble with labor, been trying to give birth for hours. The breeder brought her in at midnight and we alerted the surgeon on call. Bella had a C-section and, shortly thereafter, five healthy pups."

"Oh my, they're absolutely precious." I pick up a toasty puppy, hold him against my cheek, and smell his puppy breath. Charles Schulz was right—happiness is a warm puppy. I close my eyes, enjoying the sweet baby boxer. Newton was almost this small when we first brought him home. Holding this bundle seems to make all my cares in the world go away, if only for just a few minutes. The pup finds a warm crevice in my neck and snuggles in. The newborns in the cage make little grunting sounds as they maneuver among each other, vying for their momma's milk.

"You know, Doc, they might be looking for homes," the technician coyly suggests. "I'm just sayin'."

Her words bring me back to reality, and my wall goes up just a bit. "Tempting," I reply. "But it has to be a family decision. And besides, puppies are usually spoken for before the litter ever hits the ground."

And with that, I place the little puppy back in the cage with his mom and siblings and head down the hall to start my day, mourning for my dog.

Since our loss of Newton, it's been bittersweet any time I see a boxer as a patient. They're wonderful dogs, but at times the proximity pulls a bit too much on my heartstrings. I miss Newtie's kisses and his steadfast companionship. I even miss his slobber. Clearly, I've not fully recovered from the loss, but these darling puppies do give me something happy to ponder.

When I reach my workstation, there's a notice taped to my computer screen. It's from the ER service, and it reads: *There is an oncology case for pickup.* Hmm. This is odd. It's extremely rare for my service to acquire a case from the overnight emergency team. Though I work with serious illness, my goal is to have my patients be at home, feeling good. My technician and I head back down to ICU to see what's going on.

Callie Williams is a six-year-old Shetland sheepdog who was diagnosed with transitional cell carcinoma, the most common type of cancer arising in the bladder of a dog. She came in to see me for the first time about seven months ago, after having surgery to remove her mass. Though young for this disease, Callie has been doing well on her oral medication, which has helped keep her cancer at bay. She is given one dose per day of piroxicam, a nonsteroidal anti-inflammatory pill that can be effective against Callie's specific type of cancer. In a small percentage of cases, it can be harsh to a dog's stomach, similar to what people can experience from aspirin. But this Sheltie has been fine on this medication until now. I review her chart, and see that Callie came in last night for vomiting seven times all over Ms. Williams's white rug. From what I know of Ms. Williams, this did not make her happy. Additionally, the Sheltie has not been interested in her dog food. Ms. Williams was worried that she was sick from her treatment. Callie was admitted to the hospital and started on intravenous fluids to help rehydrate her. Meanwhile, she's been kept NPO, meaning given no food or water, to rest her stomach.

Cassidy unhooks the canine from her fluids and tries to get her out of the cage. She's a shy dog and resists big-time. She's also quite overweight, so my coworker and I both bend down to pick her up and place her on the exam table. In testing her gums and her skin turgor, I can see that she's still slightly dehydrated. With the aid of a thermometer, we know that she doesn't have a fever. When I palpate her abdomen, she splints a little in discomfort. The rest of her physical exam is unremarkable. I hold the dog still while my nurse draws the dog's blood to run some tests. On the count of three, we both lift Callie off the table and place her gently back into her cage atop a padded mat and blanket. As Cassidy hooks the dog back up to her fluids, I head to my workstation to begin writing up the Sheltie's chart.

Twenty minutes later, the results of Callie's blood work are placed in front of me. I chuckle and shake my head, thinking how easy it is to blame the cancer treatment. I reach for the phone.

"Hello, Ms. Williams? How are you this morning?" I ask.

"Fine," she offers. "But tired from all that nonsense last night. And tired from cleaning my rugs."

"I'm sorry that your girl had to spend the night in the hospital. Any chance Callie could have gotten into something?"

"Nooo, not reeeally," she says slowly, thinking.

"Could she have eaten something other than her dog food?" I prod.

"Well, yes, now that you mention it. She stole a bunch of barbecue ribs off of a plate and ate them right up. I told Tom not to leave the dish down low, but he didn't listen. Is that why she got sick?"

"Yeah, it looks like Callie has pancreatitis, which she likely got from eating rich food that wasn't her own. Thankfully, with supportive care and some medications, she'll be back to herself in no time."

"Oh, thank goodness," Ms. Williams says. "And thank you. So this has nothing to do with her cancer?"

"That's right. This is just a regular dog problem—wanting to eat something that she shouldn't."

"Can I come get her now?"

"We'll have to see how she does during the day. We need to rest her stomach. Let's touch base later this afternoon. If she's better, she can definitely go home. Otherwise, she might need one more night with us," I tell Ms. Williams. We hang up with me promising to call the concerned woman later today.

With some anti-nausea medication, intravenous fluids, pain medication, and rest, Callie will be just fine. When she's ready to go home, we'll have her owners give her a bland diet at first, gently reintroducing food to her GI tract.

I suppose we all get in our own way sometimes. For me, the rumblings in my head are what get me into trouble. I continue to work on trying to quell the noise and remind myself what deserves my energy and attention, and what doesn't. I suppose barbecue ribs aren't a bad way to get off track. The Sheltie just overdid it. I glance at myself in the reflection of a window. My arm raises; my hand strokes my hair. My brown locks have almost fully come back. I feel a bit foolish for having worried so much about my hair. But at the time, it meant a lot to me. It was the only thing I had any control over, or really the only thing I thought I had any real control over.

By afternoon, it's evident that Callie is feeling much better. She hasn't vomited since her admission to the hospital, and she's alert and watching the happenings of the ICU around her. We offer her a small amount of water, to see if she can keep it down. The Sheltie laps at it, but then sniffs around her bowl, looking for food. While my technician stays with Callie, I head down the hall to get the canine a small amount of bland dog food. When I come back, Callie is standing, wagging her tail in anticipation. She readily eats the soft diet, then looks at us as if to say, "That's it? Surely you've got more!"

"Okay, Callie, you're a good girl. We'll give you more once

we see that your stomach is okay and you keep that down." I stroke the dog on the top of her head, then close the cage door.

Callie is sent home at the end of our workday, dinnertime, which I'd guess is Callie's favorite time of the day. But Ms. Williams is given strict instructions as to what her Sheltie is and is not allowed to eat, especially over the next few days. We need to be gentle on her GI tract. The dog will continue to receive some anti-nausea medication at home. Ms. Williams will call us if she has any questions or if concerns arise.

I turn off my computer and pack up for the day. As I head out of the hospital, I find that I'm looking forward to telling my family about the boxers that were born just last night. There is nothing cuter than a little pup, but I just don't think we're ready yet to fully open our hearts to a new addition. It does beg the question, when does the grieving process end? I always tell my clients that they'll know when the time is right; perhaps I should take some of my own advice.

Months have gone by and I still have not gotten used to the house being so quiet without a four-legged friend. I find it easy to get caught up in my daily tasks and just plod along, but it's lonelier without someone following me from room to room, or eagerly greeting me as I enter the house. I do wonder about a new addition as I sit down to the computer.

"Hey, Mom!" Peter shouts as he bounds down the stairs.

"I'm in here," I call out from the kitchen.

"Guess what?!"

"Well, um—"

"I got in! I got in! I got into the University of Rochester!" In his excitement, Peter throws his arms around me and squeezes tight. A mom craves those hugs.

"Sweetheart, I am *so* proud of you!" I say, squeezing him back. "That is fantastic!"

"I got into a few others, too, but I want to go to Rochester."

"But see, you did well. You did this on your own. And, honey, it's always nice to be asked, to have options. Will you show me the email?"

"Sure, then I want to call Dad."

In my head, I thank God for this happy moment for our son. He is on his way to adulthood. Despite my family's rough year, Peter has landed just fine.

At dinner that night, Mike and I toast Peter with glasses of sparkling apple cider, the good stuff. Mike taps his glass with a fork, then clears his throat to speak.

"Ahem. Peter, we could not be any prouder of you! You've worked hard. We're so happy that you were accepted to your first-choice college, and I know that you'll do well in whatever you choose to do." Clink, clink go our three glasses.

After we begin eating, I decide to test the waters.

"Hey, guys, I've actually been doing some research about a new addition for us. Like . . . another boxer."

"I knew you were up to something," Mike says, smiling as he takes a bite of brussels sprouts.

"Like a puppy?" Peter asks.

"Well, a puppy, or maybe a rescue or adult dog. It's not always easy to find a puppy when you want one. And there are adult dogs that often need good homes."

"Hmm. But if I'm going away to college in a few months, how will it remember and love me? How 'bout we wait for a dog until I come home from school?"

"Well, you know, I bet your mom has found something she'd like to tell us about. We could get it soon so it would have time to get to know you. And you shouldn't worry—dogs always remember those they love. Besides, it would be nice to have a dog to fill the house when you're not here. It would be good for your mom and me."

"I guess we could look," Peter offers. "But it would depend."

I feel like a giddy kid again, driving with my son to go look at a boxer. It'll be an almost two-hour trek but well worth it.

Peter and I make surprisingly good time, and we arrive

early. I decide to drive around the block a few times, and after a few loops, I pull to the curb to park in front of the breeder's house.

My son asks, "Mom, is this okay?"

"Sure, we are officially right on time."

"No, I mean, is it okay to get another dog? You know, because of Newtie?"

"Oh, honey, it's just fine. Newton knew you loved him so much. But he would want you to give another dog that same love. And in a way, you're honoring him with another boxer."

"I guess."

"And we will never forget Newtie. Ever. He was such a good boy. But maybe we can give another dog a really good home, you know?"

"Well, we're not necessarily bringing her home, right?" Unbuckling his seat belt, he says, "We'll see, right?"

"Sure," I reply. And with that, we head to the front door. Peter rings the bell, and we hear a chorus of barking boxers behind the door. Music to my ears! It is clear that someone is trying to shuffle a group of dogs. When the door finally opens, there stands a single brindle boxer wiggling her short tail at record speed. Debbie, the breeder, welcomes us in.

Standing in the entryway, I look at the dog. She is a beautiful four-year-old. The stark white stripe between her eyes and her broad white chest are outlined by her darker coat. Her brown eyes dart back and forth between Peter's and mine.

She never seems to stop looking at us. It's as if she is saying "Hello! I'm here." I reach down to pet the boxer's head. Dusty has a very soft coat, though it's like trying to pet a moving target. Just as I look over at my son to try to get a read on how he's feeling, Dusty jumps up on him, placing her front paws right on his chest. Peter bends slightly, and she gives him a multitude of kisses on his face.

Peter kneels down. Dusty almost topples him over just to get the chance to sit on his lap. Joining the fun, I kneel down and am immediately greeted with kisses as well. I wipe the moisture from my face. It is clear that this girl has enough love to go around. After we've spent only a few minutes with her, it already feels as if she's ours.

"So, do you want to take her home?" the breeder asks.

"Ahhhh," I say, stalling, caught slightly off guard. I need to confer with my son. And if I'm thinking practically, we have no dog food, no collar, no leash, no dog bed . . .

After a brief discussion with Debbie about Dusty's medical history and training, I give Dusty a quick once-over and perform a physical exam. Debbie is a good breeder and has very healthy, well-adjusted dogs. I'm told that, with her second pregnancy, Dusty needed to have a difficult C-section to deliver her puppies. Debbie elected to not put her through any more litters, and Dusty's retirement works in our favor. I bend down to examine her belly. Her C-section scar is prominent. Maybe she and I have more in common than I realize. It's not so easy to go through what she and I have been through. And an older dog is harder to place in a forever home. But we moms need to stick together. I want to tell her, "Girlfriend, I got you." I pull out my checkbook, ready to make her ours. Peter gives me an inquisitive look, then nods his head in agreement.

"You really think so?" I ask him under my breath.

"Yeah, Mom. I think we should do it. I really like her." More music to my ears. I watch as Peter pets our new addition. She's calmed down. She's standing still, enjoying the love she is getting in return.

I quickly head to my car to grab my emergency leash. A well-prepared vet always carries a spare slip lead leash in case there's a stray dog on the road. Today, this leash will bring home happiness for my family.

When I get back to the breeder's house, Dusty does three rapid spins in the air to the right. She is so excited to see the leash. Her body has twisted into a circle. Pure joy! The boxer holds still just long enough for me to put the leash around her neck, then pulls us out the front door. I think Dusty knew we were her new family before we did.

Driving back home, I am a bit stunned that we are bringing home a dog after only thirty minutes. Mike surely will be surprised. But he knows me; he knows I was going to the breeder—and quite frankly it was like sending a kid into a candy store. So, it's sort of on him. I glance over at my son seated next to me. I am met with a face that is content and happy. Looking into the rearview mirror, I can see Dusty curled up into a ball, asleep in the back. A smile comes across my face.

Running through a list of things we need—dog food, a pink dog bed, new food and water bowls, plush toys—has filled our travel time. We arrive home quicker than I expect. Opening the hatch of the station wagon, Dusty readily jumps out of the back, looking up at Peter and me as if to say, "What's next?" We will give her such tender loving care. As we head into the house, Peter has a spring in his step. I take the boxer's leash, she and I following behind my son. Dusty, looking up at me, is jauntily by my side.

CONCLUSION

For now, the enemy has surrendered. Every day may not be my best day, but I am so thankful for all my days. The C word has given me pause to look at life a bit differently. How lucky I am to get this opportunity, and yet it was right under my nose the entire time—I just never stopped to see it. The patients I treat, the pets I live with, display unbridled love, acceptance, loyalty, and companionship. They live in the moment, each and every day. They help make our lives better and show us how we can make life better as well. I am not sure that I will get past how scary our own mortality is. It seems more daunting, especially the older I get. But I will no longer give the C word the power it wants. I still can't say that damn word, but from now on whenever I think of it, it will only be with a lowercase c. In this year, I have acquired more scars than I'd ever wish on anyone. I may have had to battle to get these new scars, but I wear them proudly. In the medical world, a scar is said to remodel and reorganize, getting smaller and less noticeable with time. I am hopeful that with time, my scars will be less emotionally painful, but that the good that came from them will remain.

AUTHOR'S NOTE

I absolutely love being a medical oncologist. Working to help animals feel better is my passion. The wag of a tail or a sloppy wet kiss of appreciation brings me joy. But what truly feeds me is helping pet families have one more summer or another year with their four-legged friend. To be able to sit next to a person, to hold their fear and worry and turn that into understanding and hope, is the best part of my job. I have listened to so many people tell stories about why their four-legged family member is truly so special. I am grateful for this glimpse into their world, into their struggle. And it has been my purpose to help their pet and to help them navigate the C word. It is my hope that this book will reach a wide audience to help with life and living.

ACKNOWLEDGMENTS

For most of my life, I have done nothing on social media. When I was first diagnosed with the *C* word, I realized that I did not have the strength to constantly update my friends as to my condition, my latest treatment, or how I was feeling. So, I took to writing periodic emails to them. Initially, the group was small, though it ultimately morphed into seventy-five of my "closest" friends (and family). Many would write back, providing encouragement, giving me strength. It was a lifeline to which I clung. Many would also ask, "Have you ever thought about writing a book? You should really write a book." Once treatment concluded and I no longer sent group emails, occasionally a friend would reach out and say, "You really should think about writing a book." I disregarded their suggestions until Mike and I went away for a weekend. At the hotel, a morning newspaper came to our room. It was the end of March. I read my horoscope. It said, *You should start your book today.* I was floored! Two days later I began to write and never stopped.

I am eternally grateful to my professional literary team. You are a gift from the heavens. William Patrick, your advice and encouragement were invaluable right when I needed you the most. Thank you, Shannon Welch, for taking the chance on me. I appreciate you. Sydney Rogers, I thank you for the hours pored over the manuscript, for your thoughtfulness, and for understanding my vision. You picked up seamlessly and made the manuscript better, as if you had been with me right from day one. To the incredible crew at HarperOne, especially Louise Braverman and Lucile Culver, I am indebted to your diligence, hard work, and professionalism. Thank you, Zoe Sandler, for being an important person in this big puzzle and your numerous reads. A big note of gratitude to Aileen Boyle, thank you for your many and brilliant ideas. A very big thank-you to Tina Bennett, the best literary agent a girl could ask for. I appreciate your wisdom, patience, and the work you did to help with this new chapter in my life. Without you, this book would not be. I truly value your friendship. Who knew meeting at our kids' camp many years ago would morph into where we are today? Our sons brought us together!

I would not be here if it wasn't for the medical professionals at Memorial Sloan Kettering Cancer Center. Dr. Abu-Rustum, Dr. Alektiar, Dr. Makker, I am forever grateful to you for saving my life. Dr. Pfister, your recommendations and counsel were paramount. The nursing team and support staff, thank you for putting up with me and making me feel cared for. You are invaluable to me and all of the MSKCC patients. Though not affiliated with the cancer center, Dr. Schmidt-Sarosi, thank you for being an incredible doctor. And my brother-in-law, Dr. Jeb Brown, who held my hand from near and far. I thank you.

Thank you to the Rhode Island hotel, the breathtaking Ocean House, not only for providing the newspaper that pivotal morning, but for being a safe haven where I wrote for endless hours.

To the best work team I could ever ask for, I thank you for the hours, the love, the sweat and tears. And, of course, the food and music! You were my family at the office and I cherish our memories. You made a hard job incredibly better. And you were a big reason why I came back after being on medical leave. I still always have your back, and I know you have mine. Thank you to Jenny, Shaina, Jess, Jayne, Ashleigh, JD, Courtney, Julie, Elizabeth, Jessie, Vanessa, Jodie, Crystal, Cassie, Taherrah, Tia, Purnima, Shayla, Stephanie, and Drs. Hunt, Straus, Kantrowicz, and Palescandolo—just to name a few! Thank you to the incredible veterinarians in the surrounding community. I have loved working together to help the many shared patients. A special shout-out to my PetCure Oncology work family for their incredible care of the patients, their care of the employees, and the kindnesses shown to me.

To my friends. I forever bow to you. You were and still are my crutch through life. Thank you for the numerous trips in and out of the city, the delicious meals, and your company. Sally, you went above and beyond to bring me nurturing food from your restaurant. Lisa Marie, the healing bone broth that you made was so appreciated. Angela and Jill, your steadfast friendship (and organization) were lifesaving. To those who flew across the country to visit me, Kim, Betsy, Susan, Neal, and Jeb, how can I ever say enough thank-yous? Thank you Karen, Penny, Sam A., Tracy, Amy, Mary, Colleen, Louise, Sam C., Sybil, Katy C., Stephanie, Linda, Laura, Lisa, Joanne, Marguerite, Emily and Andrew, Katy D., Grace, Wendy, Lynne, Stacy, Sung, Tina, Richard and Julie, Chris and Peggy, Angela and Phil, and Jill. I love you all.

A special note of thanks to Emily Rosenblum-Lucas, a friend and guide in the publishing process.

To Tantrum Salon, Keith and Lisa, your kindness to me meant the world. To the Pellacanis, who helped me navigate my hair loss issues, I thank you.

To Norma Rubio, for her soothing voice and healing meditations. Thank you for guiding me.

Without all of my patients and their pet parents, this book would never be. Though cancer was a sad reason for us to have met, I cherish knowing you and being trusted to try to help your beloved four-legged family members. You were the other reason I wanted to come back to work after being on medical leave. You made it all worth it. I treated your pets like my very own. I enjoyed our conversations at all of the recheck appointments. You were dedicated, vulnerable fighters and I applaud you.

To my family, despite the numerous words I have written, the times I seem to endlessly talk, I am choked up writing to you now. Mike, thank you for your love, your understanding, and for caring for me when I needed it most. It has not always been an easy ride, but I am glad that you are next to me as copilot. To my son, Peter, my "favorite." I love you endlessly, wholly and fully. You mean the world to me, and I thank God every day for you. I am incredibly proud of the person you are. And to Ramsey, my brother, thank you for the many phone calls during my treatment time. They were more comforting than you'll ever know.

Lastly, I am grateful to all of the boxers I have had along the way. By my side, they make the journey that much better. Thank you.

ABOUT THE AUTHOR

Since the age of seven, Dr. Alsarraf has wanted to be a veterinarian. As a young child, she was forever drawn to animals. Though most of her family members were physicians or nurses, Renee was determined to care for our four-legged friends. Even before attending veterinary school, Renee worked at a veterinary clinic, took riding lessons, competed in obedience trials with her boxer, Drummer, and helped special needs children ride horseback.

While at veterinary school at Michigan State University, Renee realized that many pet parents would struggle with the grief of losing their pet. This inspired Renee to create Michigan State University's Pet Loss Support Group. Led by a therapist specializing in bereavement counseling, each month sorrowful pet parents would come to better understand the grief process, to work through their feelings, and to be heard in a supportive community.

After veterinary school, Dr. Alsarraf completed an internship and a medical oncology residency in New York City at the Animal

Medical Center (AMC) in 1994. She received further radiation therapy training at AMC and worked in a tissue culture lab at Memorial Sloan Kettering Cancer Center. Since becoming board certified in medical oncology, Dr. Alsarraf has created medical oncology services in Kansas City and in New Jersey. Currently, she is a consultant for a national radiation therapy company (PetCure Oncology). Dr. Alsarraf has authored book chapters, published numerous peer-reviewed journal articles, and has spoken on the national as well as the local level.

Dr. Alsarraf lives in Montclair, New Jersey, and is married to a veterinary ophthalmologist. They have one son whom she cherishes as well as Dusty, her beloved, bossy, six-year-old female boxer. In her free time, Dr. Alsarraf likes to hunt for antiques, garden, cook, and listen to her son play piano.